Foreword

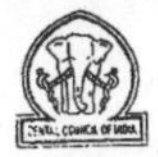

भारतीय दन्त परिषद

DENTAL COUNCIL OF INDIA

(CONSTITUTED UNDER THE DENTISTS ACT 1948)

Aiwan-E-Galib Marg, Kotla Road, New Delhi-110 002

DR. ANIL KOHLI

MDS (Lko), DNBE (USA)

President DNO-4379

Awardee:

- Padmashri
- Padmabhushan
- Dr. B.C. Roy National Award

Telephone : 23220204 Direct
23238542, 23236740
: 0091 - 11 - 23231252
: 0091 - 11 - 23220204

E-mail : dciindia@hotmail.com

Website : http://www.dciindia.org

The progressive concept is changing very fast from subjective to objective. In many universities a part of the professional examination question papers contain objective type questions.

All the competitions contain only Multiple Choice Questions (MCQs). In MCQ type objective question papers, questions from the full course can be covered, while only in subjective type question papers, it is not possible to cover the complete course of the subject, because out of an average of about 50 topics in a subject only 6 questions on 6 topics can be asked. When the question papers are of subjective type, students do only the superficial selective reading and lack the complete and deeper knowledge of the subject. With MCQ type of question papers the chances of leakage of the question papers are also very much reduced as they cover complete course of the subject and the students have to read complete course.

This book provides excellent and comprehensive coverage, covering all the aspects of the subject with unique and to the point explanations, which are in simple and easy language. This book is of great value to the students preparing for BDS, MDS and various competitive examinations.

Anil Kohli

President, Dental Council of India

Preface

This book has been written keeping professional and PG Dental Entrance Examinations in mind. Answers with the Explanations and references have been given. It has been observed that many toppers of subjective type professional university examinations do not fair well in objective type competitive examinations. This book will guide them in their preparations for objective type competitive examinations.

References are from standard books and medical dictionaries. The questions have been selected by many toppers who have got flying success in the examinations and competitions. This book will be a handy guide in preparations for examinations and competitions. The questions in this book have been compiled after analyzing almost all the question papers of recent years of all the colleges, institutes and universities conducting BDS and MDS professional estaminations and PGMEE (Dental).

The secret of success in competitive examinations lies in proper guidance and regular hard work. This book is excellent for quick revision of complete course just few days before the examinations and competitions. This book will be a great asset for the students preparing for dental professional examinations, the postgraduate dental entrance examinations, various other competitions and interviews.

In professional examinations also the trend is very fast changing towards MCQs. This book will also be very useful for the students of graduate and postgraduate courses, as it contains questions, which are usually asked in periodical assessments during graduate and postgraduate courses and in final examinations and all the competitions.

For the preparation for competitions the aim of this book is to encourage the readers to detect areas of weakness in understanding the subject matter so that they may again study the textbooks for better and comprehensive review of the subject.

Every effort has been made to update the book with recently asked questions in all the competitions, examinations and PGMEE Dental examinations. This book will be very useful for all the students for a quick revision of complete course before examinations and competitions, and will prepare them to face any examination and competition with full confidence.

Authors

Tips for Success

1. As the competitions have become very tuff, it will be better to start the preparations for MDS admission competition, the day you take admission in BDS course.

   Recent survey has shown that the students who have succeeded in PGMEE (Dental) in first attempt have started preparations for it from the day one, when they joined B.D.S. course, irrespective of their joining a government or private college. Therefore the students aiming for MDS course should start preparations for PGMEE (Dental) from the very first day of joining B.D.S. course. They must prepare all the subjects of first year, solve MCQS with the standard of PGMEE (Dental) in the first year itself. Likewise in every year they must prepare all the subjects of that year with PGMEE (Dental) standard and solve MCQs. In this way when they complete BDS course their all subjects are prepared with PGMEE (Dental) standard. After appearing in final professional examination they should crash revise all the subjects and appear with full confidence for success.
2. Start your crash preparations after relaxing for about a week after last BDS examination. If you have about one year for the PGMEE (Dental) examination divide this period of study as follows. (A) Give six months for initial preparation (revising Textbooks and solving MCQs), (B) Four months for final preparation (solving MCQs from books) and (C) Next 45 days for solving of MCQs. from question papers of similar examinations of previous 10 years, (D) In last 15 days group discussion with the students who are better than you and have secured higher ranks than you in last examinations and competitions.

   If time is less than divide the time proportionately for suggested method of preparations.

3. Procure all study material.
4. Be organized in your study.
5. Plan your study hours.
6. Understand each chapter of each subject and attempt connected MCQs before proceeding to the next chapter. If you correctly answer less than 90% of MCQs, repeat the chapter. In the same way prepare all the chapters of a subject and then only change to another subject.
7. Finish subjects one by one starting from non-clinical, then para-clinical and finally clinical subjects.
8. Consult your seniors who have passed the examinations with a good score. Follow their advice but not blindly.
9. Revise the textbooks of all the subjects thoroughly from the beginning to the end. Do not do selective reading except only in final revision.
10. Aim for the sky because you will invariably fall short and will land at the hill top i.e. aim for top position then only you will get selected in the subject and college of your choice.
11. Practice self-assessment tests and solve model test papers in the prescribed time limit, to know (i)which chapters require revision (ii) to get a feel of examination conditions and (iii) to assess your speed of solving MCQs so that you can plan your timing in the examination hall accordingly.
12. Practice, practice and practice MCQs. again and again with reasoning, no guess work
13. Observe time limit yourself while solving model test papers and examination question papers.
14. Have confidence, relax and be tension-free while attempting questions in the examination.
15. Read the questions carefully to understand them, think and then answer.

Information and Suggestions

Remember - You can do it. Always try for the top slot because if you aim for the sky, you would atleast reach the hilltop. **Remember** - You can do it and have to do it. There is no alternative.

Tentative months of various entrance exams		Approximate No. of seats available
All India PG	– Jan	158
AIIMS	– May/Nov	6
BHU	– July	6
PGI Chandigarh	– June	6
MAHE	– Jan to Feb	100
Various states/College/ University Entrance Examinations	– Jan to Dec.	3500

The following is the approximate percentage of MCQs appeared in the various postgraduate entrance examinations in previous years, and recommended weeks for revision of the subject.

Subjects for Revision	No. of MCQ's %age	Recommended Weeks for Revision	
		Textbooks	MCQ books
1. Purely preclinical	8	2	2
2. Applied preclinical	9	2	2
3. Oral and Dental Pathology & Oral Medicine	19	4	4
4. Oral and Maxillofacial Surgery	6	2	2
5. Periodontics	5	1	1
6. Prosthodontics & Dental materials	13	3	3
7. Conservative dentistry	6	2	2
8. Orthodontics	4	2	2
9. Dental Radiology	2	2	1

Contd...

Subjects for Revision	No. of MCQ's %age	Recommended Weeks for Revision	
		Textbooks	MCQ books
10. Endodontics	8	2	2
11. Community dentistry and Preventive dentistry	8	1	2
12. Gen. Medicine and Surgery	6	1	1
13. Pedodontics	4	1	1
Total	**100**	**25**	**25**

1. Only hard labour and vast knowledge are not enough but mastering the technique of taking MCQ examination is equally important.
2. First clear the basic fundamentals to have wider and better understanding of the subjects. You must read the textbooks as much as possible before taking up the books of MCQS.
3. Do not attempt the questions that you are not sure of. Negative marks due to guesswork always take you down in the merit list. Even 1 mark can change your merit tremendously, and you may loose the already secured seat.
4. If there is negative marking, it is better to leave a question rather than to attempt it wrongly. Make sure that there is no negative marking then only you may take a chance. In most of the competitions there is negative marking hence be careful and make doubly sure that there is no negative marking.
5. Research in psychology has concluded that most of us mark the right choice first and due to second thoughts mark a wrong choice
6. The entrance examinations are to test the basic fundamental knowledge of the subject. Mostly the choices are straight forward and not to trick you. Answer each question from general principles rather than from exceptions.
7. Appear in all the entrance examinations in which you are eligible. You never know when luck may favour you.
8. Work harder and harder and keep on appearing in all the entrance examinations till you succeed. Very soon you will succeed.

Contents

NOTE		
Harrison	=	*Principles of Internal Medicine, 17th Edition, Page No.*
HM P	=	*Textbook of Pathology by Harsh Mohan, 6th Edition, Page No.*
COM P	=	*Oral Medicine by Satish Chandra and Others, Page No.*
SOP P	=	*Shafer's Text Book of Oral Pathology, 6th Edition, Page No.*
T.C.M.D.	=	*Taber's Cyclopedic Medical Dictionary 21st Edition*

One

Gastrointestinal and Hepatobiliary System

QUESTIONS

1. **The most useful screening test for lead poisoning is:**
   A. Aminolaevulinic acid in urine
   B. Elevated free erythrocyte protoporhyrin (FEP)
   C. Basophilic stippling of RBCs
   D. Blood lead levels

2. **Obstructive jaundice may be seen as a side effect of therapy with:**
   A. Reserpine
   B. Furosemide
   C. Chlorpromazine
   D. Isoniazid

3. **Which does not contain CPK (creatinine phosphokinase) ?**
   A. Muscle
   B. Myocardium
   C. Liver
   D. Brain

4. **A group of people suffer form abdominal cramps, diarrhea and vomiting two hours after eating sweets. The suspected aetiological agent is:**
   A. Salmonella typhimurium
   B. Staphylococcus aureus
   C. Strepto coccus visidens
   D. Clostridium botulinum

5. **A patient having acute viral hepatitis shows increased bilirubin, transaminase and:**
   A. HBe Ag
   B. HBe Ab
   C. HBc Ag
   D. HBs Ag

6. Peptic ulcer may be associated with all of the following, except:

A. Hyperparathyroidism
B. Cirrhosis of liver
C. Pernicious anemia
D. Pulmonary emphysema

7. The following condition is associated with low serum gastrin level:

A. Gastrinoma
B. Duodenal ulcer
C. Gastric carcinoma
D. Pernicious anemia

8. Average incubation period of mumps is:

A. 1 to 5 days
B. 7 to 10 days
C. 14 to 21 days
D. 3 weeks to 3 months

9. Repeated vomiting can lead to:

A. Cheyne-Stokes respiration
B. Tetany
C. Severe metabolic alkalosis
D. All of the above

10. Sustained diarrhea can lead to:

A. Respiratory alkalosis
B. Metabolic acidosis
C. Respiratory acidosis
D. Metabolic alkalosis

11. Lymphadenopathy is seen in all except:

A. Chancroid
B. Syphilis
C. Gonorrhea
D. LGV

12. The most common complication of amoebiasis is:

A. Liver abscess
B. Lung abscess
C. Bone infection
D. Hemolytic anemia

13. Complication of peptic ulcer includes each of the following except:

A. Perforation
B. Malignant transformation
C. Pernicious anemia
D. Hemorrhage

14. All of the following are true about Wilson's disease except:
   A. Chronic active hepatitis
   B. Increase serum cetroplasmin
   C. Increase liver copper
   D. Hemolysis

15. The treatment of choice for pseudomembranous colitis is:
   A. Amikacin
   B. Ampicillin
   C. Vancomycin
   D. None of the above.

16. All of the following are true about histopathological appearance in cirrhosis except:
   A. There is nodular transformation of the lobular architecture
   B. Thrombosis is seen in the biliary blood vessels
   C. Extensive fibrosis occurs involving most of the cells
   D. Intracellular hyaline deposition occurs in alcoholics

17. A patient with episodic jaundice and conjugated hyperbilirubinemia had normal liver biopsy. The most likely diagnosis is:
   A. Criggler Najjer syndrome
   B. Dubin-Johns syndrome
   C. Rotor's syndrome
   D. Gilbert's syndrome

18. A 10 year old boy has presented with food poisoning after 24 hours of consuming food. He has passed 8 loose stools. The drug preferred in this patient is:
   A. Ciprofloxacin
   B. Metronidazole
   C. Ciprofloxacin and metronidazole combination
   D. None of the above

19. Ulcerative colitis is known to cause all of the following except:
   A. Hepatocellular carcinoma
   B. Lrities

C. Sclerosing cholangits
D. Erythema nodosum

20. Gaucher's disease, Tay- Sachs disease and Niemann-Pick disease are the examples of:
A. Protein storage diseases.
B. Glycogen storage diseases
C. Lipid storage diseases
D. None of the above

21. Vomiting of blood is known as:
A. Hematemesis
B. Epistaxis
C. Malena
D. Hereditary

22. Enzyme deficient in Tay-sachs disease is:
A. Hexosaminidase A
B. Sphingomyelinase
C. Lysosomal glucosidase
D. Glucocerebrosidase

23. Which of the following organs is most commonly and most seriously involved in amyloidosis?
A. Kidney
B. Liver
C. Spleen
D. Heart

24. Most of the absorbed lead is taken up by:
A. Blood
B. Bone
C. Liver
D. Soft tissues

25. Ethanol is mainly absorbed from:
A. Whole large intestine
B. Stomach
C. Colon
D. None of the above

26. Virchow's node is:
A. Supraperitoneal lymph node
B. Supralaryngeal lymph node
C. Supraclavicular lymph node
D. Supradiaphragamatic lymph node

27. Crohn's disease can involve:
A. Any portion of gastrointestinal tract
B. Colon only

C. Small intestine and color
D. Large intestine

28. Most serious complication of ulcerative colitis is:
A. Malabsorption syndrome
B. Bleeding
C. Colon carcinoma
D. None of the above

29. Biochemical diagnosis of Wilson's disease is based on:
A. Decrease in hepatic copper content
B. Decrease in serum ceruloplasmin
C. Decrease in urinary excretion of copper
D. All of the above

30. Amyloid material can be best diagnosed by:
A. Polarized microscopy
B. X-ray crystallography
C. Scaning electron microscopy
D. Electromicroscopy

31. Which of the following is not an example of massive splenomegaly:
A. Chronic myeloid leukemia
B. Chronic malaria
C. Tropical splenomegaly
D. Acute lymphoblastic leukemia

ANSWERS AND EXPLANATIONS WITH REFERENCES

1. B. *Ref:* HM P–240 & T.C.M.D.
- Lead poisoning may occur in children or adults due to accidental or occupational ingestion. –HM
- Lead poisoning, chronic ingestion or inhalation of lead, damaging the central and peripheral nervous systems, the blood-forming organs, and the gastro-intestinal tract. Early symptoms include loss of appetite, weight loss,

anemia, vomiting, fatigue, weakness, headache, lead line on gums, apathy or irritability, and a metallic taste in the mouth. Later, symptoms of paralysis, sensory loss, incoordinnation and vague pains develop. Laboratory diagnosis is made through evidence of anemia; blood lead level above 5 ug/dl; elevated free erythrocyte protoporphyrin (FEP); increased excretion of lead in urine; characteristic X-ray changes in the ends of growing bones.

2. **C.** *Ref:* HM P–596, COM P–167 & T.C.M.D

- Jaundice or icterus refers to the yellow pigmentation of the skin or sclerae by bilirubin.
- Jaundice results from excess of billrubin in the circulation. Jaundice manifests as yellow discoloration of skin, oral mucous membrane and sclera when the serum billrubin exceeds 2 to 3 mg/dl. Jaundice may be caused by destruction of red blood cells (Hemolytic jaundice), obstruction of bile duct (obstructive jaundice) or due to hepatic diseases (hepatocellular jaundice)–COM
- Chlorpromazine is a tranquilizing agent used primarily in its hydrochloride form in major and minor psychotic states. Trade name for chlorpromazine hydrochloride is Emetial.

3. **C.** *Ref:* HM P–296

- Creatinine phosphokinase (CPK) exist as three isoenzymes in human tissues:
  A. CPK-1 or CPK–BB: Found in BRAIN.
  B. CPK-2 or CPK–MB: Found in MYOCARDIUM
  C. CPK-3 or CPK–MM: Found in SKELETAL MUSCLE
- Thus creatinine phosphokinase is absent in LIVER but is found in all above mentioned site.

4. **B.** *Ref:* T.C.M.D

- Staphylococcus aureus is a species of gram-positive, coagulase-positive anaerobes commonly present on the skin and mucous membranes, esp. those of the nose and mouth, characterized by the production of a golden-yellow pigment. It causes suppurative conditions such as boils, carbuncles, and internal abscesses in humans. Various strains of this species produce toxins including those that cause food poisoning, staphylococcal scalded skin syndrome, and toxic shock syndrome. Some strains also produce hemolysins and staphylokinase.

5. **D.** *Ref:* Harrison P–1822-1844, HM P– 607 & COM–103

- "After a person is infected with HBV, the first virologic marker detectable in serum is HbS Ag. Circulating HBs Ag precedes elevations of serum aminotransferase activity and clinical symptoms and remains detectable during the entire icteric or symptomatic phase of acute hepatitis B and beyond." Harrison's P–1823
- HBsAg may also be demonstrated in the cell membrane of hepatocytes of carries and chronic hepatitis patients by Orcein staining (orange positivity) but not in the hepatocytes during acute stage of illness. –HM
- Hepatitis D is caused by the hepatitis delta virus, a defective RNA virus that requires HBsAg to replicate. The acute Hepatitis D occurs in two following forms :
  A. As a coinfection with acute Hepatitis B, which is usually self-limiting.
  B. As a superinfection in chronic hepatitis B carrier.– COM

6. **C.** *Ref:* HM P–549 & COM P–166, 200

Peptic ulcers are the areas of degeneration and necrosis of gastrointestinal mucosa exposed to acid-peptic secretions. – HM

- The peptic ulcers in the gastrointestinal tract are most frequently caused by infections with Helicobacter pylori and use of non-steroidal anti-inflammatory drugs.

Pernicious anemia is caused by vitamin B12 deficiency. It is caused due to failure of vitamin B12 due to atrophy of gastric mucosa resulting in lack of secretion of intrinsic factor.– COM

- Associated diseases with Peptic ulcer
  A. Some patients with multiple endocrine adenomatosis, type I (MEA I) present with gastrin-secreting tumors. This probably accounts for the reported association of duodenal ulcer disease with hyperparathyroidism.
  B. Antral atrophic gastritis may be caused by back-diffusion of bile through the pylorus and is associated with a high incidence of gastric ulcers.
  C. Patients with rheumatoid arthritis have an increased risk of ulcer disease, which probably is secondary to the drugs used for treatment.
  D. Chronic obstructive pulmonary disease has been found in a significant number of gastric ulcer patients; cirrhosis of the liver and chronic renal failure are demonstrated in a significant number of duodenal ulcer patients.

7. **C.** *Ref:* HM P–555 & T.C.M.D.
- Carcinoma of the stomach comprises more than 90% of all gastric malignancies and is the leading cause of cancer-related deaths in countries where is incidence is high. –HM
- Gastric cancer is diagnosed by barium radiography of the GI tract with fluoroscopy, fiberoptic endoscope gastroscopy and biopsy, and gastric acid stimulation testing. Studies to rule out specific organ metastases include computed tomography scans, chest radiographs, liver and bone scans, and liver biopsy.

8. **C.** *Ref:* Harrison P–1220, HM P–533 & COM P–128
- Mumps is an acute, systemic, communicable viral infection whose most distinctive feature is swelling of one or both parotid glands.
- The most common inflammatory lesion of the salivary glands particularly of the parotid glands, is mumps occurring in children of school-age.–HM
- Mumps is an acute contagious viral infection caused by

a ribonucleic acid (RNA) Paramyxovirus. It mostly affects the salivary gland, but may also involve gonads. It predominantly occurs among children and young adults. The incubation period of infection is 2 to 3 weeks. It is transmitted by direct contact with droplets of saliva.–COM

- Mumps is an acute contagious paramyxovirus disease seen mainly in childhood, involving chiefly the salivary glands, most often the parotids, but other tissues, e.g., the meanings and testes (in postpubertal males), may be affected.

9. **D.** *Ref:* Harrison P–294

- This is primarily directed at correcting the underlying stimulus for HCO_3 - generation.
- In vomiting there is loss of acids leading to metabolic alkalosis, which can cause tetany and typical Cheyne-stokes respiration (also seen in diabetes).

10. **B.** *Ref:* Harrison P–247 & HM P–104

- Diarrhea is loosely defined as passage of abnormally liquid or unformed stools at an increased frequency.
- A fall in the blood pH due to metabolic component is brought about by fall of bicarbonate level and excess of H+ ions in the blood. –HM
- In diarrhea, alkalies /bases are lost from GIT leading to metabolic acidosis.

11. **C.** *Ref:* Harrison P–914, HM P–344 & COM P–209

- Angioimmunoblastic lymphadenopathy is characterised by diffuse hyperplasia of immunoblasts rather than paracortical hyperplasia only, and there is proliferation of blood vessels. The condition occurs in elderly patients with generalized lymph node enlargement and hypergammaglobulinaaemia.
- Gonorrhea is a sexually transmitted infection (STI) of epithelium and commonly manifests as cervicitis, urethritis, proctitis, and conjunctivitis.
- Gonorrhea is caused by gram-negative bacteria Neis-

seria gonorrhea. Initial infection occurs on genitourinary, rectal and orpharyngeal surfaces. – COM

- Generalized lymphadenopathy and fatigue are the classic signs of infectious mononucleosis.

12. **A.** *Ref:* Harrison P–1275 & HM P–188

- Amebiasis is an infection with the intestinal protozoan Entamoeba histolytica. About 90% of infections are asymptomatic, and the remaining 10% produce a spectrum of clinical syndromes ranging from dysentery to abscesses of the liver or other organs.
- Amoebic liver abscess may be formed by invasion of the radicle of the portal vein by thropzoites. Amoebic liver abscess may be single or multiple. The amoebic abscess contains yellowish- grey amorphous liquid material trophozoites are identified at the junction of the viable and necrotic tissue.– HM
- Intestinal amoebiasis commonly involves the cecum, ascending colon and the rectosigmoid region. The pathogens are carried by the portal vein to the liver where abscess formation may occur.

13. **C.** *Ref:* Harrison P–646, HM P–549 & COM P–166, 200

- Pernicious anemia (PA) may be defined as a severe lack of IF due to gastric atrophy.
  Ref Q. 16
  Ref Q. 16–COM
- Pernicious anemia is a type of macrocytic anemia because of vitamin B12 and folate deficiency. Blood loss from peptic ulcer usually causes normocytic normochromic anemia.

14. **B.** *Ref:* Harrison P–1981 & HM P–628

- Wilson's disease is an inherited disorder of copper homeostasis first described in 1912.
  Refer Q. 70
- Wilson's disease is an autosomal recessive disease characterized by excessive copper deposition, which, if untreated, may lead to fulminant hepatic failure.

Copper also is deposited in the brain, kidney, and cornea, which causes Kayser-Fleischer rings. CNS disease may be prominent if the diagnosis is made in adulthood. Diagnosis is suggested by decreased serum ceruloplasmin levels and is confirmed by an increased hepatic copper concentration in a liver biopsy sample.

15. **C.** *Ref:* HM P–144

- Pseudomembranous is inflammatory response of mucous surface (oral, respiratory, bowel) to toxins of diphtheria or irritant gases. –HM
- The first step in treatment is to discontinue unnecessary antibiotics, which results in improvement in most patients. Cholestyramine may be used to bind the toxin. The organism is sensitive to vancomycin, bacitracin, and metronidazole.

16. **B.** *Ref:* Harrison P–1971, HM P–618 and T.C.M.D.

- Cirrhosis is a condition that is defined histopathologically and has a variety of clinical manifestations and complications, some of which can be life-threatening.
- Cirrhosis of the liver is one of the ten leading causes of death in the western world. –Hm

17. **C.** Ref: Harrison P–263, HM P–601 and TMD

- Elevated conjugated hyperbillirubinemia is found in two rare inherited conditions: Dubin-Johnson syndrome and Rotor's syndrome. Patients with both conditions present with asymptomatic jaundice, typically in the second generation of life. The defect in Dubin-Johnson syndrome is mutations in the gene for multiple drug resistance protein 2. These patients have altered excretion of billrubin into the bile ducts. Rotor's syndrome seems to be a problem with the hepatic storage of billrubin. Differentiating between these syndromes is possible, but clinically unnecessary, due to their benign nature.
- Rotor's syndrome is another form of familial conjugated hyperbillrubinaemia with mild chronic jaundice but

differs from Dubin-Johnson syndrome in having no brown pigment in the liver cells. The disease is inherited as an autosomal recessive character. – HM

- Rotor syndrome is an inherited liver disorder that is transmitted as an autosomal recessive trait; it is similar to but genetically distinct from Dubin-Johnson syndrome.
- Rotor's syndrome is a rare autosomal recessive condition.
- Cirrhosis is a chronic disease of the liver marked by formation of dense perilobular connective tissue, degenerative changes in the parenchymal cells, structural alteration of the cords of liver lobules, fatty and cellular infiltration, and sometimes development of areas of regeneration.

18. C. *Ref:* Harrison P–855 & H.M. P–474

- Metrondiazole, a synthetic imidazole, is active only against bacteria and protozoa. The reduction of metronidazole's nitro group by the bacterial anaerobic electron-transport system produces a transient series of reactive intermediates that are thought to cause DNA damage.
- Metronidazole has broad spectrum cidal activity against protozoa, including Giardia Lamblia in addition to the above two. Many anaerobic bacteria, such as Bact. fragilis, Fusobacterium, Clostridium perfringens, anaerobic Streptococci and the helminth Dracunculus medinensis are sensitive. It does not affect aerobic bacteria. Clinically significant resistance has not developed among the parasites for which it is used. Clinically combination gives best results.

19. A. Ref: Harrison P–580, HM P–567, 633 & COM P–169

- Hepatocellular carcinoma (HCC) is one of the most common malignancies worldwide. Most HCC patients have two liver diseases, cirrhosis and HCC, each of which is an independent cause of death.

- Classically ulcerative colitis begins in the rectum, and in continuity extends upwards into the sigmoid colon, descending colon, transverse colon, and sometimes may involve the entire colon. Hepatocellular carcinoma (HCC) or liver cell carcinoma, also termed as hepatoma, is the most common primary malignant tumour of the liver. –HM
- Ulcerative colitis is a chronic inflammatory disease of mucosa and submucous of the colon. It is characterized by abdominal pain, rectal bleeding and diarrhea. It frequently causes anemia, hypoproteinemia and electrolyte imbalance. -COM
- Carcinoma of the colon is associated with long-standing disease of great extent (usually pancolitis).

20. C. *Ref:* Harrison P–2455, HM P–262 &TMD

- Gaucher disease is an autosomal recessive disorder that results from defective activity of acid β-glycosidase; >250 mutations have been described at the GBA locus of such patients.
- Gaucher's disease is an autosomal recessive disorder in which there is mutation in lysosomal enzyme, acid β-glucosidase (earlier called glucocerebrosidase), which normally cleaves glucose from cermide.
- Niemann-Pick Disease is also an autosomal recessive disorder characterised by accumulation of sphingo-myelin and cholesterol due to defect in acid sphingo-myelinase. –HM
- Gaucher's disease is a chronic congenital disorder of lipid metabolism caused by a deficiency of the enzyme beta-glucocerebrosidace.
- Tay-Sachs disease is an inherited disease transmitted as an autosomal recessive trait.
- Niemann-Pick disease is a disturbance of sphingolipid metabolism characterized by enlargements of liver and spleen, anemia, lymphadenopathy and progressive mental and physical deterioration.

21. A. *Ref:* Harrison P- 242, HM P–539 & TMD

- Hematemesis raises suspicion of an ulcer, malignancy, or Mallory-Weiss tear, whereas feculent emesis is noted with distal intestinal or colonic obstruction.
- Massive hematemesis (vomiting of blood) may occur due to vascular lesions in the oesophagus.– HM
- Hematemesis is the vomiting of blood and the blood is often clotted and mixed of food, subsequent stool may be tarry.

22. A. *Ref:* Harrison P–2453 & TMD

- About 1 in 30 Ashkenazi Jews is a carrier for Tay-Sachs disease, which is caused by total hexosaminidase A (Hex A) deficiency.
- Tay-sachs disease is an inherited disease transmitted as an autosomal recessive traits it is because of the lack of the enzyme Hexosaminidase A, which is important in sphingolipid metabolism, sphingolipid accumulate in the cells, esp. those of the nerves and the brain.

23. A. *Ref:* Harrison P–2145, HM P–82, COM P–94 & TMD

- Amyloidosis is a term for diseases that are due to the extracellular deposition of insoluble protein fibrils in tissues and organs.
- Amyloidosis is the term used for a group of disease characterised by extracellular of fibrillar preoteinaceous substance called amyloid having common morphological appearance, staining properties and physical structure but with variable protein (or biochemical) composition. – HM
- Amyloid deposits frequently occur in oral cavity. They appear as waxy deposits on lips, gingival and tongue and lead to macroglossia and gross enlargement of oral tissues. – COM
- Amyloid resembling starch; Starchlike. Amyloidosis is a metabolic disorder marked by amyloid deposits in organs and tissues.

24. **B.** *Ref:* HM P- 240 & TMD

- Bones, teeth, nails and hair representing relatively harmless pool of lead. About 90% of absorbed lead accumulates in the developing metaphysic of bones in children and appears as areas of increased bone densities ('lead lines') on X-ray. Lead lines are also seen in the gingiva.– HM
- Lead is a conductor attached to an electrocardiograph .Lead is a metallic element whose compounds are poisonous; atomic weight 207.2, atomic number 82, specific gravity 11.35.

25. **B.** *Ref:* HM P- 160 &TMD

- Absorption of alcohol begins in the stomach and small intestine and appears in blood shortly after ingestion. Alcohol is then distributed to different organs and body fluids proportionate to the blood levels of alcohol. – HM
- Ethanol is a colorless, volatile, flammable liquid .Its molecular weight is 46.07 C. It is present in fermented or distilled liquor and is obtained, in its pure form, from grain fermentation and fractionation distillation.

26. **C.** *Ref:* Harrison P–266, HM P–200 and TMD

- A carefully executed general physical examination can yield valuable clues concerning the etiology of abdominal swelling. Thus palmar erythema and spider angiomas suggest an underlying cirrhosis, while supraclavicular adenopathy (Virchow's node)should raise the question of an underlying gastrointestinal malignancy
- Virchow's lymph node is nodal metastasis preferentially to supraclavicular lymph node from cancers of abdominal organs e.g. cancer stomach, colon, and gall bladder. –HM
- Virchow's node is enlargement of one of the supraclavicular lymph nodes; usually indicative of primary carcinoma of thoracic or abdominal organs.

27. A. *Ref:* HM P–565 &TMD

- Crohn's disease or Regional enteritis is an idiopathic chronic ulcerative IBD, characterised by transmural, non-caseating granulomatous inflammation, affecting most commonly the segment of terminal ileum and/or colon, through any part of the gastrointestinal tract may be involved. – HM
- Crohn's disease is the term for a number of chronic inflammatory disease of the gastrointestinal tract, it is ulcerative colitis and regional ileitis or enteritis.

28. C. *Ref:* Harrison P–1886, HM P–565, COM P–169 & TMD
Refer Q. 114

- Ulcerative Colitis is a mucosal disease that usually involves the reaction and extends proximally to involve all or part of the colon.
- Ulcerative Colitis is an idiopathic form of acute and chronic ulcero-inflammantory colitis affecting chiefly the mucosa and submucousa of the rectum and descending colon, though sometime it may involve the entire length of the large bowel. –HM
- The major clinical symptoms of ulcerative colitis are bloody diarrhea and abdominal pain. In severe cases, signs of arthritis and liver disease also may be present. A major complication of severe ulcerative colitis is toxic megacolon.

29. B. *Ref:* Harrison P–1981, HM P–628 andaTMD
Refer Q. 70

- Wilson's disease is an inherited disorder of copper homeostasis first described in 1912.
- Wilson's disease is a hereditary syndrome transmitted as an autosomal recessive trait in which a decrease of ceruloplasmin permits accumulation of copper in various organs (brain, kidney, liver and cornea) associated with increased intestinal absorption of copper.

30. A. *Ref:* HM P–82, COM P–94
Refer Q. 153

- By H & E staining under light microscopy,amyloid appears as extracellulal, homogeneous, structureless and eosinophilic hyaline material; it stains positive with Congo red staining and shows apple-green birefringence on polarizing microscopy. –HM

Diagnosis of amyloidosis

i. Biopsy
ii. Fine needle aspiration of abdominal subcutaneous fat followed by congo- red staining and polarizing microscopic examination is acceptable and useful technique with excellent results.
iii. Injection of congo red dye intravenously in living patient.
iv. Other test like electrophoresis, bone marrow aspiration.

31. D. *Ref:* Harrison P–692 and HM P–387

- The treatment of patients with precursor B cell ALL (Acute lymphoblastic leukemia) involves remission induction with combination chemotherapy, a consolidation phase that includes administration of high-dose systemic therapy and treatment to eliminate disease in the CNS, and a period of continuing therapy to prevent relapse and effect cure.
- Massive enlargement in splenomegaly (below umbilicus) occurs in CML, myeloid metaplasia with myelofibrosis, storage diseases, thalassaemia major, chronic malaria, leishmaniasis and portal vein obstruction. –HM
- Splenomegaly of moderate grade is seen in acute leukemia, while massive splenomegaly is seen in chronic leukemias.

Two

Hematological System

QUESTIONS

1. Haemophilia A is characterized by the presence of following features, except:

A. Prolonged partial thromboplastin time
B. Low factors VIII levels
C. Bleeding into soft tissues, muscles & joints
D. Prolonged prothrombin time

2. Normal hemoglobin is:

A. Hemoglobin M
B. Hemoglobin H
C. Hemoglobin S
D. Hemoglobin A

3. In anemia of chronic disorders following increase/s:

A. Serum Fe
B. Ferritin
C. None of the above
D. Both of the above

4. Lymphadenopathy is seen in all except:

A. Chancroid
B. Syphilis
C. Gonorrhea
D. LGV

5. Earliest change seen in iron deficiency anemia is:

A. Decreased serum iron
B. Increased serum ferritin
C. Decreased serum transferrin
D. Decreased serum ferritin

6. True regarding methemoglobinemia is:

A. Amyl nitrite is used in the treatment of symptomatic cases
B. Hemoglobin is in the ferrous from

C. Levels greater then 5% are almost always fatal
D. Oxygen saturation is normal

7. A person vaccinated with hepatitis B will present with the following markers in the blood:
A. Anti-HbeAg B. Anti-HBV
C. 1gGAnti-HBV D. Anti-HbsAg1gM

8. All of the following changes are seen in hemolytic anemia except:
A. Increased reticulocyte count
B. Increased haptoglobin ?
C. Increased hemoglobinuria
D. Iron deficiency

9. A patient with hemolytic anemia, jaundice and pigmented gall stones. The most likely diagnosis is:
A. Sickle cell anemia
B. Iron deficiency anemia
C. Thalassemia major
D. Hereditary spherocytosis

10. Edema (Oedema) tends to appear when plasma albumin is reduced to a level of:
A. 2.5 gm/100 ml B. 25 gm/100 ml
C. 0.025 gm/100 ml D. 0.25 gm/100 ml

11. Milroy's disease is caused by abnormal development of:
A. Lymphatic vessels B. Veins
C. Arteries D. All of the above

12. Active hyperemia is characterized by:
A. Dilated arteriole B. Dilated capillaries
C. Dilated artery D. Both B. and C.

13. Which of the followings is/are an example of coagulation defects?
A. Hypofibrinogenemia B. Hypoprothrombinemia
C. Afibrinogenemia D. All of the above

14. Pin point hemorrhage is also known as:
A. Ecchymosis B. Purpura
C. Thrombus D. Petechiae

15. Marfan syndrome shows:
A. Quantitative defects in fibrillin
B. Qualitative defects in fibrillin
C. Both of the above
D. None of the above

16. Bruton's disease is:
A. X-linked hypogammaglobulinemia
B. X-linked agammaglobulinemia
C. X-linked afibrinogenemia
D. Non sexlinked agammaglobulinemia

17. Which of the following blood dyscrasias is/are caused by penicillin?
A. Thrombocytopenia B. Hemolytic anemia
C. Both of the above D. None of the above

18. In kwashiorkor-like protein energy malnutrition serum albumin level falls to:
A. Less than 2.1 gm/dl B. Less than 1.4 gm/dl
C. Less than 2.8 gm/dl D. Less than 2.5 gm/dl

19. Which of the followings is not a clinical manifestation of primary hyperaldosteronism?
A. Low level of serum renin
B. Hyperkalemia
C. Hypertension
D. None of the above

20. To the hemophilic patient which of the following should not be given:
A. Platelet factor B. Cryoprecipitate
C. EACA D. Factor VIII concentrate

21. In megaloblastic anemia the cells are:
A. Macrocytic hyperchromic
B. Macrocytic hypochromic
C. Macrocytic normochromic
D. Macrocytic hypochromic

22. Autoimmune haemolytic anemia is seen in:
A. CLL B. CML
C. AML D. ALL

23. Reduced number of platelet is found in all the condition except:
   A. Von-Willebran's disease
   B. Aplastic anemia
   C. Disseminated intravascular coagulation
   D. Acute-myelocytic leukemia

24. Christmas disease is due to deficiency of:
   A. Factor X
   B. Factor VIII
   C. Factor IX
   D. Factor V

25. Glucose -6 phosphate dehydrogenase deficiency causes:
   A. Aplastic anemia
   B. Haemolytic anemia
   C. Haemophilia
   D. Megaloblastic anemia

26. Reliable screening test for haemophilia is:
   A. CBP
   B. B T
   C. P T
   D. APTT

27. Leucocytosis is seen in:
   A. Megaloblastic anemia
   B. Steroids
   C. Blood transfusion
   D. Dengue

28. In sickle cell anemia there is substitution of :
   A. Valine for glutamic acid at the sixth position of beta chain
   B. Phenylalanine for glutamic acid
   C. Tyrosine for valine at the 6th position at beta chain
   D. All of the above

ANSWERS AND EXPLANATIONS WITH REFERENCES

1. D. *Ref:* HM P–335, COM P–204 & T.C.M.D.
   - Patients of hemophilia suffer from bleeding for hours or days after the injury. The clinical severity of the disease correlates well with plasma level of factor VIII activity. Haemophillic bleeding can involve any organ but occurs most commonly as recurrent painful

haemarthroses and muscles haematomas, and sometime as haematuria.– HM

- Hemophilia A is caused by deficiency of factor VIII, the antithemophilic factor. It is inherited as a sex-linked recessive trait that affects males. Females are clinically normal carriers. Severe bleeding occurs when factor VIII is less than 1% of normal. Factor (F) VIII levels between 1% to 7% of the normal lead to moderate bleeding. Mild symptoms such as prolonged bleeding after tooth extraction or severe trauma may occur when levels are between 7% and 50% of normal. – COM
- Hemophilia is due to a deficiency of blood coagulation factor VIII. Hemophilia is a hereditary blood disease marked by greatly prolonged coagulation time, with consequent failure of the blood to clot and abnormal bleeding, sometimes accompanied by swelling of the joints. It is a sex-linked trait transmitted by normal heterozygous females who carry the recessive gene and occurring almost exclusively in males. There are two main types of hemophilia, A and B; a third type of hemophilia C, is rare. The cause of hemophilia is deficiency of a factor in plasma necessary for blood coagulation. The term hemophilia has been used to designate a variety of blood coagulation disorders. It should be used to refer to conditions in which a specific coagulation factor is lacking.

2. D. *Ref:* Harrison P–635

- Different Hemoglobins are produced during embryonic, fetal, and adult life.
- "The tetrameric structures of common hemoglobin's are as follows: HBA (NORMAL adult hemoglobin) = 2 2: HBF (Fetal hemoglobin) 2 2; HBs (Sickle cell hemoglobin) = 2 S2; and HbA2 (a minor adult hemoglobin) = 2 2."

3. D. *Ref:* Harrison P–629 & HM P–301

- Within the erythroid cell, iron excesses of the amount needed for hemoglobin synthesis binds to a storage protein, apoferritin, forming ferritin. This mechanism of iron exchange also takes place in other cells of the body expressing transferring receptors, especially liver parenchymal cells where the iron can be incorporated into heme-containing enzymes or stored.

- Sideroblastic anemias usually show the following haematological features:
  1. There is generally usually moderate to severe degree of anemia.
  2. The blood picture shows hypochromic anemia which may be microcytic, or there may be some normocytic red cells as well (dimorphic).
  3. Absolute values (MCV, MCH and MCHC) are reduced in hereditary type but MCV is often raised in acquired type.
  4. Bone marrow examination shows erythroid hyperplasia with usually macronormoblastic erythropoiesis. Marrow iron stores are raised and pathognomonic ring sideroblasts are present.
  5. Serum ferritin levels are raised.
  6. Serum iron is usually raised with almost complete saturation of TIBC.
  7. There is increased iron deposition in the tissue. – HM
- Anemia associated with chronic inflammation is of moderate degree and reveals slight hypochromia and microcytosis. The mean corpuscular volume (MCV) is 80 to 85 3, and the mean corpuscular hemoglobin concentration (MCHC) is 30 percent to 32 percent. If stained, the marrow reveals plentiful iron stores. Also, ferritin usually is normal or only slightly elevated. Serum iron is lowered as is the total iron-binding capacity, which is unlike the clinical situation with iron deficiency anemia.

4. B. *Ref:* T.C.M.D

- Pulse Pressure is the difference between systolic and diastolic pressures. It characterizes the tone of the arterial walls. The systolic pressure is normally about 40 points greater than the diastolic. A pulse pressure over 50 points or under 30 points is considered abnormal.

5. D. *Ref:* Harrison P–629, HM P–301 & COM P–199

- Within the erythroid cell, iron excesses of the amount needed for hemoglobin synthesis binds to a storage protein, apoferritin, forming ferritin. This mechanism of iron exchange also takes place in other cells of the body expressing transferring receptors, especially liver parenchymal cells where the iron can be incorporated into heme-containing enzymes or stored.
  Refer Q. 46
- Iron-deficiency anemia (microcytic hypochromic anemia) is the most common of all anemias. It may result due to following factors:
  a. Chronic blood loss as in menstrual or menopausal bleeding, bleeding hemorrhoids or bleeding ulcer in gastrointestinal tract.
  b. Impaired absorption of iron as in partial or complete gastrectomy or in malabsorption syndrome.
  c. Inadequately dietary intake of iron.– COM
- Anemia associated with chronic inflammation is of moderate degree and reveals slight hypochromia and microcytosis. The mean corpuscular volume (MCV) is 80 to 85 3, and the mean corpuscular hemoglobin concentration (MCHC) is 30 percent to 32 percent. If stained, the marrow reveals plentiful iron stores. Also, ferritin usually is normal or only slightly elevated. Serum iron is lowered as is the total iron-binding capacity, which is unlike the clinical situation with iron deficiency anemia.

6. D. *Ref:* Harrison P–640

- Methemoglobinemias is generated by oxidation of the heme iron moieties to the ferric state, causing a characteristics bluish-brown muddy color resembling cyanosis. Mathemglobin has such high oxygen affinity that virtually no oxygen is delivered.

- Methemoglobinemia is the presence of methemoglobin in the circulating blood when severe, there is inadequate oxygenation of the tissues.

7. C. Ref: Harrison P–1932

- Hepatitis B virus is a DNA virus with a remarkably compact genomic structure; despite its small, circular, 3200-bp size, HBV DNA codes for four sets of viral products with a complex, multiparticle structure.
- Hepatitis B is a DNA virus transmitted parenterally. Individuals at high risk include in travenous drug abusers, homosexual men, and those exposed to blood and blood products.

8. B. Ref: HM P–310 &T.C.M.D.

- Haemolytic anemias are defined as anemias from an increase in the rate of red cell destruction. Normally, effected cells undergo lysis at the end of their lifespan of 120 30 days within the cells of reticuloendothelial (RE) system in the spleen and elsewhere (extravascular haemolysis), and haemoglobin is not liberated into the plasma in appreciable amounts. – HM
- Hemolytic anemia resulting from hemolysis of red blood cells; may be congenital or may be caused by the effects of toxic agents or by severe pre-eclampsia.

9. C. *Ref:* Harrison P–640, HM P–323 & COM P–201

- The thalassemia syndromes are inherited disorders of α - or β-globin biosynthesis.
- β–thalassemia major, also termed Mediterranean or Cooley's anemia is the most common form of congenital haemolytic anemia.
- Clinical features: Clinical manifestations appear insidiously and are as under:
  1. Anemia starts appearing within the first 4-6 months of life when the switch over from γ-chain to β-chain production occurs.
  2. Marked hepatosplenomegaly occurs due to excessive red cell destruction, extramedullary haematopoiesis and iron overload.

3. Expansion of bones occurs due to marked erythroid hyperplasia leading to thalssemic facies and malocclusion of the jaw.
4. Iron overload. – HM

- β-thalassemia major is the most severe form of thalassemia. Hemoglobin level may reach below 2 to 3 g/dl with hematocrit less than 20. There is extensive hemolysis.– COM
- Thalassmias are genetic disorders characterized by diminished synthesis of the globin chains.

10. A. *Ref:* Harrison P–233, HM P–97 & TMD
Refer Q. 121

- The displacement of fluid into a limb may occur at the expense of the blood volume in the remainder of the body, thereby reducing effective arterial blood volume and leading to the retention of NaCl and H_0O until the deficit in plasma volume has been corrected.
- Edema may result from increased permeability of the capillary walls; increased capillary pressure due to venous obstruction or heart failure; lymphatic obstruction; disturbance in renal function etc.

11. A. *Ref:* HM P–97 & TMD

- Milroy's disease or hereditary lymphoedema is due to abnormal development of lymphatic channels. It is seen in families and the oedema is mainly confined to one or both the lower limbs.– HM
- The lymphatic vessel carries lymph toward a subclavian vein. Plasma that leaves capillaries and become tissue fluid is collected by lymph capillaries.

12. D. *Ref:* HM P–105 & TMD

- The dilatation of arteries, arterioles and capillaries is effected either through sympathetic neurogenic mechanism or via the release of vasoactive substances. The affected tissue or organ is pink or red in appearance (erythema). – HM
- Hyperemia is a form of macula; red areas of the skin that disappear on pressure. Active hyperemia caused by increased blood flow.

13. D. *Ref:* Harrison P–363, HM P–335 & TMD

- The human hemostatic system provides a natural balance between procoagulant and anticoagulant forces. The procoagulant forces include platelet adhesion and aggregation and fibrin clot formation; anticoagulant forces include the natural inhibitors of coagulation and fibrinolysis.
- Instead of spontaneous appearance of petechiae and purpuras, the plasma coagulation defects manifest more often in the form of large ecchymoses, haematomas and bleeding into muscles, joints, body cavities, GIT and urinary tract.– HM
- Hypoprothrombinemia is a deficiency of blood clotting factor II (prothrombin) in the blood.
- Hypofibrinogenemia is decreased fibrinogen in the blood.
- Afibrinogenemia is a rare blood disease marked by an absence or decreased of fibrinogen in the blood plasma so that the blood is incoagulable; may be congenital or acquired.

14. D. *Ref:* HM P–331, COM P–79 & TMD

- Vascular bleeding disorders, also called non-thrombocytopenic purpuras or vascular purpuras, are normally mild and characterised by petechiae, purpuras or echymoses cofined to the skin and mucous membrane. -HM
- Petechiae are the very minute purplish red hemorrhagic spots of pinpoint to pinhead size, which are not blanched by pressure. They are less than 2 mm in diameter. – COM
- Petechia is a small, purplish, hemorrhagic spot on the skin that appears in certain severe fever and in indicative of great prostration, as in typhus.

15. C. *Ref:* Harrison P–2468 & TMD

- Marfan syndrome features that primarily affect the skeleton, the cardiovascular system, and the eyes.
- Marfan's Syndrome is a hereditary condition of connective tissues, bones, muscles, ligaments and skeletal structures.

16. B. *Ref:* Harrison P–2058 & TMD

- Mutations of Bruton's tyrosine kinase (Btk) gene are responsible for X-linked agammaglobulinemia.
- Agammaglobulinemia is a broad term pertaining to disorder marked by an almost complete lack of immunoglobulins or antibodies.

17. C. *Ref:* COM P–204, 200 & TMD

- The most common acquired platelet disorders are idiopathic thrombocytopenia purpura (ITP) and thrombotic thrombocytopenia purpura (ITP).

  Hemolytic anemia occurs due to excessive destruction of red blood corpuscles. Factors responsible for destruction of erythrocytes may be classified into intracorpuscular defects and extracorpuscular factors. – COM
- Dyscrasia is an old term meaning abnormal mixture of the four humors. The word is now used as a synonym for disease. Penicillin is a group of antibiotics biosynthesized by several species of molds, esp. Penicillin notatum and P. chrysogenum.

18. C. *Ref:* HM P–246 & TMD

- Kwashiorkor which is related to protein deficiency though calorie intake may be sufficient. –HM
- Kwashiorkor is a severe protein-deficiency type of malnutrition of children. It occurs after the child is weaned.

19. B. *Ref:* Harrison P–283, HM P–798 & TMD

- Hyperkalemia, defined as a plasma K+ concertration >5.0 mmol/L, occurs as a result of either K^+ release from cells or decreased renal loss.
- Cohn's syndrome (Primary hyperaldosteronism) is more frequent in adult females. Its principal features are as under:
  1. Hypertension, usually mild to moderatew diastolic hypertension.

2. Hypokalaemia and associated muscular weakness, peripheral neuropathy and cardiac arrhythmias.
3. Retention of sodium and water.
4. Polyuria and polydipsia due to reduced concentrating power of the renal tubules. –HM

- Hyperkalemia is an excessive amount of potassium in the blood. This condition is usually caused by inadequate excretion of potassium or the shift of potassium from tissues.

20. B. *Ref:* Harrison P–710, HM P–340, COM P–204

- Cryoprecipitate is a source of fibrinogen, factor VIII, and von Willebrand factor (vWF). It is ideal for supplying fibrinogen to the volume-sensitive patient.
- Cryoprecipitate is a source of insoluble plasma proteins, fibrinogen, factor VIII and vWF. Indications for transfusion of cryoprecipitate are for patients requiring fibrinogen, factor VIII and vWF. Transfusion of single unit of cryoprecipitate yields about 80 IU of factor VIII. –HM
- Concentrates for treatment of hemophilia A (F VIII) and B (F IX) deficiencies are specific for each type of hemophilia. Therefore a correct diagnosis is a must for effective replacement therapy. –COM

21. C. *Ref*: Harrison P–643 & HM P–294

- The megaloblastic anemias are a group of disorders characterized by the presence of distinctive morphologic appearances of the developing red cells in the bone marrow.
- Macrocytic: MCV is raised e.g. in megaloblastic anemia due to deficiency of vitamin B12 or folic acid. –HM
  - i. Macrocytic hypochromic
    - MCV (Mean volume) and
    - MCH (Mean) MCHC are reduced
    - Eg Iron deficiency anemia, thalessimia, sideroblastic anemia. (Normocytic normochromic)
    - MCV MCH MCHC are normal

Hematological System

- Eg Hemolytic, aplastic anemia, acute blood loss, anemia of chronic disease.

ii. Macrocytic normochromic
   - MCV is raised
   - Eg Megaloblastic anemia.

22. **A**. *Ref:* Harrison P–659, HM P–312

- Except for countries where malaria is endemic, AIHA is the most common form of acquired hemolytic anemia.
- Conditions predisposing to Autoimmune Haemolytic Anemia (AIHA) are as follows.

A. Warm Antibody AIHA
   1. Idiopathic (primary)
   2. Lymphomas-leukaemias e.g. non-Hodgkin's lymphoma, CLL, Hodgkin's disease
   3. Collagen vascular diseases e.g. SLE
   4. Drugs e.g. methyldopa, penicillin, quinidine group
   5. Post-viral

B. Cold Antibody AIHA
   1. Cold agglutinin disease
      a. Acute: Mycoplasma infection, infectious mononucleosis
      b. Chronic: Idiopathic, lymphomas
   2. PCH (Mycoplasma infection, viral flu, measles, mumps, syphilis) –HM

- Autoimmune haemolytic anemia occurs due to antibody production by the body against its own red cells. Depending upon the reaction to autoantibody, autoimmune haemolytic anemia is of two types.

A. "Warm antibody" autoimmune haemolytic anemia in which the auto antibodies are reactive at body temperature (37°C)

   Examples:
   - Idiopathic
   - Lymphoma, leukemias like non-Hodgkins lymphoma, Hodgkins lymphoma, CLL
   - Collegen vascular disease

- Drugs like penicillin, quinidine group, methyl dopa.
- Post viral

B. Cold antibody autoimmume haemolytic anemia in which the auto antibodies are reactive at 40C.

Examples:
- Idiopathic
- Cold agglutinin disease
- Acute condition like mycoplasma infection, infectious mononucleosis
- Chronic condition like lymphoma.
- Post viral.

23. **A.** *Ref:* Harrison P–366, HM P–336 & COM P–204

- Mucosal bleeding symptoms are more suggestive of underlying platelet disorders or von Willebrand disease (vWD), termed disorders of primary hemostasis or platelet plug formation.
- von Willebrand's disease (vWD) is the most common hereditary coagulation disorder occurring due to qualitative or quantitative defect in von Willebrand's factor. – HM
- von Willebrand's disease (vWD) is caused due to defect in factor VIII protein complex. Both males and females are affected. There is prolonged bleeding time but normal platelet count. –COM

von - Willebrand`s disease

a. It occurs due to qualitative defect in von-Willebrand`s factor (VWF).

b. VWF helps in adhesion of platelets to sub-endothelial collegen and circulates as "factor VIII - VWF" in blood.

c. The disease is characterized by normal platelet count, but the bleeding time is prolonged due to defective platelet aggregation and reduced factor VIII activity.

24. **C.** *Ref:* HM P–336 & COM P–204

- Hemophilia A or classic hemophilia occurs due to deficiency of factor VIII. Normal hemostasis requires 25 percent factor VIII activity and becomes symptomatic when the factor VIII levels are below 25 percent.

- Hemophilia B or Christmas disease is due to deficiency of factor IX.
- Hemophilia is a hereditary coagulation disorder inherited as a sex (X- linked) recessive trait.
- It is manifested clinically in males, while females are carrier.
- Inherited deficiency of factor IX (Christmas factor or plasma thromboplastin component) produces Christmas disease or hemophilia B.
- Hemophilia B is caused due to deficiency of factor IX (Christmas factor) plasma thrombplastin component.

25. B. *Ref:* HM P–310

– Haemolytic anemias are defined as anemias resulting from an increase in the rate of red cell destruction. Normally, effected cells undergo lysis at the end of their lifespan of 120 30 days within the cells of reticuloendothelial (RE) system in the spleen and elsewhere (extravascular haemolysis), and hemoglobin is not liberated into the plasma in appreciable amounts. –HM

i. The Red blood cells are protected against oxidation due to generation of reduced glutathione.
ii. In a person with G6PD deficiency fails to develop sufficient amount of reduced glutathione in their red cells, so there is oxidation occurs and haemoglobin precipitates within red cells and "HEINZ BODIES" formed.
iii. Glucose -6- phosphate dehydrogenase is an enzyme required for hexose monophosphate shunt for glucose metabolism.

26. D. *Ref:* HM P–335 & COM P–204

i. Acquired partial thromboplastin time or partial thromboplastin time measures the intrinsic system factor as well as factor common to both intrinsic and extrinsic systems (factor X, V, VIII, prothrombin, fibrinogen. *Example:* Heparin therepy liver disease disseminated intravascular coagulation are common cause of long PTT.

ii. Prothrombin time measures the extrinsic factor VII as well as factors in the common pathway (factor X, V, VIII, prothrombin fibrinogen).

- Normal prothrombin time is 10 to 14 second.
  Example: Vitamin K deficiency, warfarin therepy, liver disease and disseminated intravasculartion.
- Classic Hemophilia (Hemophilia A)

Laboratory Findings

1. Whole blood coagulation time is prolonged in severe cases only.
2. Prothrombin time is usually normal.
3. Activated partial thrombplastin time (APTT or PTTK) is typically prolonged.
4. Specify assay for factor VIII shows lowered activity. The diagnosis of female carrier is made by the findings of about half the activity of factor VIII, while the manifest disease is associated with factor VIII activity below 25%. –HM
   Refer Q. 208.–COM

27. **B**. *Ref:* HM P–145

- Leucocytosis commonly accompanies the acute inflammatory reactions, usually in the range of 15,000-20,000/l. When the counts are higher than this with 'shift to left' of myeloid cells, the blood picture is described as leukaemoid reaction. –HM
  a. Lab finding in dengue includes leucopenia, thrombocytopenia and in many cases elevation of serum aminotransferase.
  b. In megaloblastic anemia, diagnostic features are leucopenia with hypersegmented granulocyte and mild to moderate thrombocytopenia.
  c. The earliest change in peripheral blood after acute blood loss is leucocytosis.
  d. After a single dose of glucocorticoids the circulating concentration of neutrophils increases while the lymphocytes, monocytes, eosinophils, basophils in the circulation decreases. The increase in neutrophils

is due to both the increased influx into the blood from the bone marrow and decreased migration from the blood vessels, leading to a reduction in the number of cells at the site of inflammation.

e. The reduction in circulating lymphocytes, monocytes, eosinophils, and basophils is primarily the result of their movement from the vascular bed to lymphoid tissue.

28. **A.** *Ref:* Harrison P-637, HM P-318 & COM P–201

- Most patients with sickling syndromes suffer from hemolytic anemia, with hematocrits from 15-30%, and significant reticulocytosis. Anemia was once thought to exert protective effects against vasoocclusion by reducing blood viscosity.
- Sickle cell anemia (SS) is a homozygous state of HbS in the red cells in which an abnormal gene is inherited from each parent. – HM
- Sickle cell anemia is an autosomal recessive anemia characterized by sickle shaped erythrocytes which lead to stasis and hemolysis of the red cells. The sickling of erythrocytes is due to lower oxygen tension or increased blood pH. –COM
- Thalassemia and sickle cell anemia are combinedly known as haemoglobinopathies.In sickle cell anemia, the red blood cells contain sickle hemoglobin (Hbs) which develop sickling whenever they are exposed to lower oxygen tension.

Three

Cardiovascular System

QUESTIONS

1. Fluid therapy in a patient of shock should begin with:

A. Lomodex infusion
B. Crystalloid infusion
C. Blood transfusion
D. Plasma transfusion

2. The following can mimick the physical signs of mitral stenosis:

A. Primary pulmonary hypertension
B. Atrial septal defect
C. Ventricular septal defect
D. Left atrial myxoma

3. The investigation of choice for diagnosis of pericardial effusion is:

A. Echocardiography
B. CO_2 angiography
C. Computed tomography
D. Magnetic resonance imaging

4. The most common form of hypertension (HT) is:

A. Essential HT
B. Endocrinal HT
C. Renovascular HT
D. Systolic HT

5. The most common cause of right ventricular failure is:

A. Aortic stenosis
B. Mitral stenosis
C. Pulmonary embolism
D. Secondary to left ventricular failure

6. Best physical sign which characterises mitral stenosis is:
A. Third heart sound (S3)
B. Pulsatile liver
C. Soft, single second heart sound (S2)
D. Loud first heart sound (S1)

7. Aspirin is given in M.I. because it:
A. Inhibits thromboxane
B. Inhibits cytokines
C. Inhibits interleukins
D. Stops bleeding

8. In which condition cardiac failure does not occur in infants:
A. Anemia B. Supravalvular
C. Coarctation of aorta D. ASD

9. Most common cause of mitral stenosis in child is:
A. Congenital
B. Rheumatic heart disease
C. Papillary dysfunction
D. Infective endocarditis

10. In mitral stenosis what is seen:
A. Right ventricular hypertrophy
B. Left ventricular hypertrophy
C. Left arterial hypertrophy
D. Right arterial hypertrophy

11. Pain in angina pectoris is caused by:
A. Moderate use of alcohol
B. Inadequate blood supply to the heart
C. Hypertension
D. Diabetes mellitus

12. Drug contraindicated in Ventricular fibrillation is:
A. Digoxin B. Propranolol
C. Phenylephrine D. All of the above

13. Drug of choice in right ventricular infarct is:

A. Diuretic B. Digitalis
C. Vasodilator D. Fluid i.v.

14. A male healthy 70 years old person all of a sudden become repeatedly unconscious for only few seconds five times in 24 hours without any other discomfort. Most likely management includes:

A. Angioplasty B. Pace maker
C. Both of the above D. None of the above

15. Which of the followings is/are a form of coronary heart disease(s) ?

A. Myocardial infarction
B. Angina pectoris
C. Atherosclerotic heart disease
D. All of the above

16. In heart failure, fluid in the peritoneum is:

A. Exudate B. Transudate
C. Both of the above D. None of the above

17. Widespread edematous involvement of subcutaneous tissue is known as:

A. Congestion B. Ascitis
C. Anasarca D. Hyperemia

18. Which of the followings produce (s) generalized edema?

A. Severe infections
B. Anaphylactic reactions
C. Anoxia
D. All of the above

19. Cardiogenic shock can occurs in:

A. Aortic value dysfunction
B. Cardiac tamponade
C. Myocardial infarction
D. All of the above

20. Thrombi mostly occurs in:
A. Arteries of lower extremities
B. Veins of lower extremities
C. Arteries of upper extremities
D. Veins of upper extremities

21. Thrombi which do not cause complete obstruction of a vessel lumen are known as:
A. Mural thrombi
B. Occlusive thrombi
C. Both of the above
D. None of the above

22. Mural thrombi are commonly found in:
A. Heart chambers
B. Arteries
C. Lymphatic vessels
D. Veins

23. Lines of Zahn are feature of:
A. Antemortem thrombus
B. Postmortem clot
C. Both of the above
D. None of the above

24. Which of the followings is not a feature of antemortem thrombus?
A. It does not produce vessel distension
B. It is white and red
C. It is dry and friable
D. It is adherent to endothelium

25. Most significant complication of venous embolism is:
A. Obstruction of pulmonary artery
B. Obstruction of aorta
C. Obstruction of pulmonary vein circulation
D. None of the above

26. Fat embolism occurs in:
A. Bone fractures
B. Trauma to adipose tissue
C. Chronic alcoholism
D. All of the above

27. In which of the following organs infarct formation is rare?

A. Liver
B. Brain
C. Lung
D. Both B. and C.

28. Which of the followings causes(s) sudden cardiac death?

A. Coronary atherosclerosis
B. Mitral value prolapse
C. Endocarditis
D. All of the above

29. Most common cause of chronic cor pulmonale is :

A. Wegener's granulomatosis
B. Chronic obstructive lung disease
C. Metabolic acidosis
D. Cystic fibrosis

30. Chronic cor pulmonale is characterized by:

A. Hypertrophy of right ventricle
B. Hypertrophy of right atrium
C. Both A. and B.
D. Dilatation of right ventricle

31. Which of the following conditions increase(s) the risk of infective endocarditis?

A. Prosthetic heart valves
B. Preexisting cardiac abnormalities
C. Intravenous drug abuse
D. All of the above

32. Which of the followings is not included in tetralogy of Fallot?

A. Right atrial hypertrophy
B. Overriding of aorta
C. Right ventricular flow obstruction
D. Ventricular septal defect

33. Which of the followings is not a hemodynamic consequence of tetrology of Fallot?
A. Decreased blood flow to the lungs
B. Right-to -left shunting
C. Increased blood flow through the aorta
D. None of the above

34. Serous pericardial effusion is found in:
A. Blunt chest trauma
B. Malignancy
C. Mediastinal lymphatic obstruction
D. Congestive heart failure

35. Most common malignancy in heart is:
A. Angiosarcoma
B. Rhabdomyosarcoma
C. Myxoma
D. Secondaries of primary tumors of other organs

36. Cyanosis is found in case of:
A. Right to left shunts
B. Transposition of the great vessels
C. Tetralogy of Fallot
D. All of the above

37. Diastolic pressure in full-blown syndrome of malignant hypertension is:
A. Greater than 120 mm Hg
B. Less than 120 mm Hg
C. Greater than 140 mm Hg
D. Greater than 160 mm Hg

38. All of the following are typically associated with the loss of 40 percent of the circulating blood volume except:
A. A decrease in the heart rate
B. A decrease in the central venous pressure.
C. A decrease in the blood pressure
D. A decrease in the urine output.

39. Schilling test is performed to find out:
A. Poncreatic enzyme deficiency
B. B12 malabsorption
C. Folic acid level
D. Coronary artery disease

40. Left side heart failure results in:
A. Oedema of lungs B. Oedema of spleen
C. Oedema of legs D. Oedema of liver

41. After myocardial infarction all the following enzymes levels are high except:
A. Serum glutamic oxaloacetic
B. Lactate dehydrogenase (LDH)
C. Creatine phosphokinase (CPK)
D. Serum ornithine carbamyl transferase (SOCT)

42. White infarcts occur in one of the following organ:
A. Ovary B. Lung
C. Intestine D. Heart

43. Characteristic of rheumatic heart disease is:
A. Aschoff bodies B. Apoptotic bodies
C. Chromaffin bodies D. Pea nodules

ANSWERS AND EXPLANATIONS WITH REFERENCES

1. B. *Ref:* HM P–111 & TMD
- Compensated shock is achieved by activation of various neuro-hormonal mechanisms causing widespread vasoconstriction and by fluid conservation by the kidney. –HM
- Crystallized infusion is steeping a substance in hot or cold crystal like water in order to obtain its active principal.

2. D. *Ref:* Harrison P–1576 & HM P–450
- Pulmonary hypertension, an abnormal elevation in

pulmonary artery pressure, may be the result of left heart failure, pulmonary parenchymal or vascular disease, thromboembolism, or a combination of these factors.

- Mitral insufficiency is caused by RHD in about 50% of patients but in contrast to mitral stenosis, pure mitral insufficiency occurs more often in men (75%).–HM
- Left-sided failure. Dyspnea on exertion, orthopnea, and paroxysmal nocturnal dyspnea occur due to reduced left ventricular output and increased left atrial pressure. In mitral stenosis the symptoms of left ventricular failure usually are not due to left ventricular dysfunction but, rather, to the mitral stenosis itself.

3. A. *Ref:* HM P–457 & T.C.M.D.

- Accumulation of fluid in the pericardial cavity due to non- inflammatory causes is called hydropericardium or pericardial effusion. – HM
- Pericardial effusion is the inflammation caused by acute pericarditis often produces exudation of fluid into the pericardial space. When fluid accumulates slowly the pericardium expands to accommodate it. When fluid accumulates rapidly, however, it compresses the heart and thus, inhibits cardiac filling. This latter condition is known as cardiac tamponade.
- Echocardiography is a noninvasive diagnostic method that uses ultrasound to visualize internal cardiac structures. All cardiac valves can be visualized, and the dimensions of each ventricle and the left atrium can be measured.

4. A. *Ref:* Harrison P–1549 & COM P–153

- Essential hypertension in which the causes of increase in blood pressure is unknown. Essential hypertension constitutes about 80-95% patients of hypertension.–HM
- Primary or Essential or Idiopathic Hypertension: The cause is unknown. It is mostly found in those individuals

who are working under stress, tension, hurry and worry. –COM

- Hypertensions doubles the risk of cardiovascular disease, including coronary heart disease (CHD), congestive heart failure (CHF), ischemic and hemorrhagic stroke, renal failure, and peripheral arterial disease.
- Essential HT form about 90% of cases of hypertension, followed by about 8% Renovascular HT.

5. D. *Ref:* Harrison P–1705

- Although transient hypotension is common in patients with RV infraction and inferior MI, persistent CS due to RV failure accounts for only 3% of CS complicating MI.
- When LVF occurs, the filling pressure in the left ventricle becomes elevated, increasing the work load on the right ventricle. Thus overtaxed, the right ventricle eventually also fails.

6. D. *Ref:* Harrison P–1465 & HM P–450

- Rheumatic fever is the leading cause of mitral stenosis (MS).
  Refer Q. 26.
- The mitral valve remains open during most of diastole due to the pressure gradient across the stenotic mitral value in mitral stenosis. Ventricular systole then closes the valve forcibly with a resulting loud S1 sound.

7. A. Ref: HM P–450
Refer Q 26

- Aspirin is a widely used analgesic, antipyretic, and anti-inflammatory agent; also used as an antiplatelet agent. Syn acetylsalicylic acid.

8. C. *Ref:* Harrison P–1462, HM P–687, COM P–157 & T.C.M.D.

- Narrowing or constriction of the lumen of the aorta anywhere along its length but is most common distal to the origin of the left subclavian artery near the insertion of the ligamentum arteriosum.

- Coarctation of the aorta causes systolic hypertension in the upper part of the body due to constriction itself. Diastolic hypertension results from changes in circulation. –HM
- Coarctation of aorta is characterized by narrowing of the aortic arch distal to origin of the left subclavian artery. –COM
- Coarctation of aorta is a localized malformation resulting in narrowing of the aorta.

9. **B.** *Ref:* HM P–450 & COM P

- All the causes of mitral stenosis may produce mitral insufficiency, RHD being the most common cause. – HM
- Rheumatic heart disease of childhood that mostly occurs between six to sixteen years of age. It is caused by group A beta hemolytic streptococcal infection. This infection causes lesions in the joints, heart, nervous system and subcutaneous tissues. –COM
- Rheumatic heart disease is aortic insufficiency usually is present to some degree in most cases of rheumatic heart disease. While mitral stenosis usually predominates, aortic insufficiency occasionally is the most severe lesion seen in this disease.

10. **A.** *Ref:* HM P–450
Refer Q. 26

- In the mitral stenosis the right ventricle must generate enough force both to overcome the resistance offered by the stenotic valve and to propel blood through constricted pulmonary arteries. Pulmonary arterial pressure may increase to three to five times the normal level, eventually resulting in right ventricular failure.

11. **B.** *Ref:* Harrison–87 & HM P–429

- The primary cause for pain in angina pectoris is the inadequate blood supply to the heart.

- Angina pectoris is a clinical syndrome of IHD resulting from transient myocardial ischaemia. It is characterised by paraoxysmal pain in the substernal or precordial region of the chest which is aggravated by an increase in the demand of the heart and relieved by a decrease in the work of the heart. – HM

12. A. Ref: HM P–455

- Idiopathic restrictive (Obliterative or Infiltrative) Cardiomyopathy form of cardiomyopathy is characterised by restriction in ventricular filling due to reduction in the volume of the ventricles. –HM
- Digoxin is a cardioactive steroid glycoside obtained from Digitalis lanata. Largely eliminated by the kidneys.

13. B. *Ref:* TMD

- These are glycosidic drugs having cardiotonic property. Cardiotonic drugs increase myocardial contractility and output in a hypodynamic heart, without a corresponding increase in O_2 consumption. Thus, myocardial efficiency is increased.
- Digitalis is the dried leaves of Digitalis Purpurea used in powered form in tablets or capsules.

14. B. *Ref:* Harrison P–1416 & COM P–158

- Permanent pacemaking is the only reliable therapy for symptomatic fatigue, exercise bradycardia in the absence of extrinsic and reversible etiologies such as increased vagal tone, hypoxia, hypothermia, and drugs.
- Permanent pacemaker are used in various cardiac diseases. These disease include the following:
  1. Heart failure.
  2. Symptomatic heart block and bradycardia
  3. Brady-tacky syndrome
  4. Carotid hypersensitivity
  5. Neurocardiogenic syncope
  6. Hypertrophic cardiomyopathy – COM

- Most likely there is conduction defects hence pace maker is required.

15. **D.** *Ref:* TMD

- Narrowing of the coronary arteries sufficient to prevent adequate blood supply to the myocardium either basal oxygen needs are unmet or the oxygen supply is insufficient to meet any increased demand, as in work.

16. **B.** *Ref:* HM P–96 & TMD

- The oedema may be of 2 main types:
  1. Localised when limited to an organ or limb e.g. lymphatic oedema, inflammatory oedema, allergic oedema.
  2. Generalised (anasarca or dropsy) when it is systemic in distribution, particularly noticeable in the subcutaneous tissues e.g. renal oedema, cardiac oedema, nutritional oedema.

     Besides, there are a few special forms of oedema (e.g. pulmonary oedema, cerebal oedema. Depending upon fluid composition, oedema fluid may be:

     A. transulate which is more often the case, such as in oedema of cardiac and renal disease; or

     B. exudates such as in inflammatory oedema.– HM
- Transudate is the fluid that passes through a membrane, esp. that which passes through capillary walls. Compared to an exudate, a transudate has fewer cellular elements and is of a lower specific gravity.

17. **C.** *Ref:* Harrison P–231, HM P–96 & TMD

- Anascara refers to gross, generalized edema. Ascites and hydrothorax refer to accumulation of excess fluid in the peritoneal and pleural cavities, respectively, and are considered to be special forms of edema.

  Refer Q. 118

- Anasarca is a generalized infiltration of edema fluid into subcutaneous connective tissue.

18. **D.** *Ref:* Harrison P–231, HM P–97 & TMD

- Edema is defined as a clinically apparent increase in the interstitial fluid volume, which may expend by several liters before the abnormality is evident.
- Hypoproteinaemia usually produces generlised oedema (anasarca). Out of the various plasma proteins, albumin has four times higher plasma oncotic pressure than globulin; thus it is mainly hypoalbuminaemia (albumin below 2.5 g/dl) that results in oedema more often. – HM
- A local or generalized condition in which the body tissues contain an excessive amount of tissue fluid is called generalized edema.

19. **D.** *Ref:* Harrison P–1702, HM P–109, COM P–17 & TMD

- Cardiogenic shock (CS) is characterized by systemic hypoperfusion due to severe depression of the cardiac depression of the cardiac index [<2.2 (L/min)/m^2] and sustained systolic arterial hypotension (<90 mm Hg), despite an elevated filling pressure [pulmonary capillary edge pressure (PCWP)>18 mm Hg].
- Acute circulatory failure with sudden fall in cardiac output from acute diseases of the heart without actual reduction of blood volume (normvolaemia) results in cardiogenic shock.–HM
- Cardiogenic shock results from severe fall in cardiac output secondary to acute diseases of heart. The commonest cause is myocardial infraction. Other conditions include rupture of value, cardiac arrhythmias, and pulmonary embolism. –COM
- Cardiogenic shock is a shock resulting from failure to maintain the blood supply to the circulatory system and tissues because of inadequate cardiac output.

20. **B.** *Ref:* HM P–118 & TMD

Table 1: Distinguishing Features of Antemortem Thrombi and Postmortem Clots

Feature	*Antemortem Thrombi*	*Postmortem Clots:*
1. Gross	Dry, granular, firm and friable	Gelatinous, soft and rubbery
2. Relation to vessel wall	Adherent to the vessel wall	Weakly attached to the vessel wall
3. Shape	May or may not fit their vascular contours	Take the shape of vessel or its bifurcation
4. Microscopy	The surface contains apparent lines of Zahn	The surface is 'chicken fat' yellow covering the underlying red 'current jelly'

- Thrombus is a blood clot that obstructs a blood vessel or a cavity of the heart. Anticoagulant is used in prevention and treatment of this condition.

21. **A.** *Ref:* TMD
- A thrombus attached to the wall of a vessel or the heart is called Mural thrombi.

22. **A.** *Ref:* TMD
- A thrombus attached to the wall of a vessel or the heart is called Mural thrombi.

23. **A.** *Ref:* TMD
- A clot formed in the heart or large vessel before death is called Antemortem thrombus.

24. **A.** *Ref:* TMD
- A clot formed in the heart or large vessel before death is called Antemortem thrombus.

25. **A.** *Ref:* TMD
- An obstruction of the pulmonary artery or one of its branches, usually caused by an embolus from thrombosis in a lower extremity is called pulmonary embolism.

26. D. *Ref:* TMD

- Fat embolism is an embolism caused by globules of fat obstruction blood vessels. It frequently occurs after fracture of long and pelvic bones and may cause dissemination intravascular coagulation.

27. D. *Ref:* TMD

- An area of tissue in organ or part that undergoes necrosis following cessation of the blood supply, this may result from occlusion or stenosis of the supplying artery or, more rarely, from occlusion of the veins that drains the tissue.

28. D. *Ref:* HM P–428, COM P–154 & TMD

- The term acute coronary syndromes include a triad of acute myocardial infarction, unstable angina and sudden cardiac death. – HM
- Causes of coronary heart diseases are as follows:
  a. Coronary atherosclerosis
  b. Aortic valvular disease
  c. Coronary embolism
  d. Coronary arterial spasm
  e. Dissecting aneurysm
  f. Vasculitis
  g. Carbon monoxide poisioning
  h. Techycardia
  i. Acute anemia – COM
- Mitral value prolapse is a common and occasionally serious condition in which the cusp or cusps of the mitral valve prolapse into the left atrium during systole.
- Endocarditis is an inflammation of the lining membrane of the heart, It is usually confined to the covering of a valve and some times to the lining membrane of the chamber.

29. B. *Ref:* HM P–438 & TMD

- Chronic cor pulmonale is more common and is often preceded by chronic pulmonary hypertension. Following chronic lung diseases can cause chronic pulmonary hypertension and subsequent cor pulmonale:

1. Chronic emphysema
2. Chronic bronchitis
3. Pulmonary tuberculosis
4. Pneumoconiosis
5. Cystic fibrosis
6. Hyperventilation in marked obesity (Pickwickian syndrome)
7. Multiple organised pulmonary emboli. – HM

- Chronic corpulmonale disease process that decreases the ability of the lungs to perform ventilation. Diseases that cause this condition are chronic bronchitis, pulmonary emphysema, chronic asthma, and chronic bronchiolitis, also called chronic obstructive lung disease.

30. C. *Ref:* TMD

- Chronic corpulmonale's diagnostic criteria include a history of persistent dyspnea on exertion with or without chronic cough, and less than half of normal predicted maximum breathing capacity.

31. **D.** *Ref:* HM P–445

- Infective or bacterial endocarditis (IE or BE) is serious infection of the valvular and mural endocardium caused by different forms of microorganisms and is characterised by typical infected and friable vegetations. – HM
- Myocarditis is an acute interstitial myocarditis of unknown cause, the endocardium and pericardium being unaffected.

32. **A.** *Ref:* HM P- 425, COM P–157 & TMD

- Tetralogy of Fallot is the most common cyanotic congenital heart disease, found in about 10% of children with anomalies of the heart. –HM
  Refer Q. 35–COM
- Tetralogy of Fallot is an anomaly of the heart consisting of (a) pulmonary stenosis, (b) inventricular septal defect, (c) dextroposed aorta that receives blood from both ventricles, and (d) hypertrophy of the right ventricle.

33. **D.** *Ref:* HM P– 425, COM P–157 &TMD

Refer Q. 172

Refer Q. 35-COM

- Pericarditis is an inflammation of the pericardium, this condition may be caused by tuberculosis, mycoses, infection by pyogenic organisms, collagen disease, uremia, myocardial infarction, neoplasms or trauma.

34. **D.** *Ref:* HM P–419, COM P–155 & TMD

- The term congestive heart failure (CHF) is used for the chronic form of heart failure in which the patient has evidence of congestion of peripheral circulation and of lungs. CHF is the end-result of various forms of serious heart disease. –HM
- Congestive heart failure refers to inadequacy of the heart to pump enough blood to meet the metabolic demands of the body. –COM
- Pericardial is the membranous fibroserous sac enclosing the heart and the bases of the great vessels. Serous pericardial is the parietal and visceral pericardial membranes.

35. **D.** *Ref:* HM P–459 &TMD

- Metastatic tumours of the heart are more common than the primary tumours. About 10% cases with disseminated cancer have metastases in the heart. Most of these result from haematogenous or lymphatic spread. In descending order of frequency, primary sites of origin are: carcinoma of the lung, breast, malignant lymphoma, leukaemia and malignant melanoma.– HM
- Malignancy is a neoplasm or tumor that is cancerous as an opposed to benign.

36. **D.** *Ref:* Harrison P–230, COM P–157 &TMD

- Cyanosis refers to bluish color of the skin and mucous membranes resulting from an increased quantity of reduced hemoglobin, or of hemoglobin derivatives, in the small blood vessels of those areas.

Refer Q. 35. – COM

- Cyanosis is slightly bluish, grayish, slate like or dark purple discoloration of the skin caused by the presence of abnormal amounts of reduced hemoglobin in the blood.

37. A. *Ref:* HM P–685, TMD

- Hypertension is a common disease in industrialized countries accounts for 6% of death worldwide.
- According to the criteria, normal cut-off values for systolic and diastolic blood pressure are taken as <120 and <80 mmHg respectively. –HM
- Malignant hypertension is a form of hypertension that progresses rapidly, accompanied by severe vascular damage. It may progress to the point of death.

38. A. *Ref:* Harrison P–1418, HM P–93

- Failure to increase the heart rate with exercise is referred to as chronotropic incompetence. This is alternatively defined as a failure to reach 85% of predicted maximal heart rate at peak exercise, or failure to achieve a heart rate>100 beats/min with exercise or a maximal heart rate with exercise less than two standard deviations below that of an agematched control population.
- Intravascular fluid or blood plasma comprises about 5% of the body weight. Thus plasma content is about 3 liters of fluid out of 5 liters of total blood volume. –HM
- Normally the patient in shock develops unconsciousness, weakness, pale, cold, clammy limbs, weak pulse, low blood pressure, oligouria (fluid conservation by kidney) and tachycardia.

39. B. *Ref:* Harrison P-643 & HM P–308

- Two mechanisms exist for cobalamin absorption. One is passive, occurring equally through buccal, duodenal, and ileal mucosa; it is rapid but extremely inefficient, <1% of an oral dose being absorbed by this process.
- Schilling test is done to detect vitamin B12 deficiency as well as to distinguish and detect lack of IF and mala-

bsorption syndrome. The result of test also depend upon good renal function and proper urinary collection. –HM

i. Schiller's test – Carcinoma of cervix
ii. Schilling test – Vitamin 12 malabsorption
iii. Rosewaller test – Rheumatoid arthritis
iv. Paul- Bunnel test – Infectious mononucleosis
v. The substance used in SICKLING TEST is sodium metabisulfite.
vi. Kveim's test – Sarcoidosis

40. A. *Ref:* HM P–419

- The clinical manifestations of left-sided heart failure result from decreased left ventricular output and hence there is accumulation of fluid upstream in the lungs. –HM
- Left heart failure - oedema of lungs
- Right heart failure - Generalised oedema involving, spleen, liver, kidney etc.

41. D. *Ref:* Harrison P–1443 & HM P–434, 314

- Heart failure (HF) is a clinical syndrome that occurs in patients who, because of an inherited or acquired abnormality of cardiac structure and/or function, develop a constellation of clinical symptoms (dyspnea and fatigue) and signs (edema and rales) that lead to frequent hospitalizations, a poor quality of life, and a shortened life expectancy.
- Certain proteins and enzymes are released into the blood from necrotic heart muscle after acute MI. Measurement of their levels in serum is helpful in making a diagnosis and plan management.–HM
- SGOT, MB fraction of CPK and LDH are the enzymes in MI, they serve as cardiac markers and help in diagnosis and treatment plan.
- The estimation of CPK2 isoenzyme is the earliest indicator of MI. SGOT is the second enzyme to rise in myocardial infarction (24 to 36 hours).

- LDH levels begin after 24 hours and reaches peak in 3 to 6 days, and returns to normal in 14 days.

42. D. *Ref:* HM P–430

- Infarcts are most frequently located in the left ventricle. Right ventricle is less susceptible to infarction due to its thin wall, having less metabolic requirements and is thus adequately nourished by the thebesian vessles. – HM

Infarct Location

i. Red or haemorrhagic infarcts Lungs and intestine
ii. Pale or white infarcts Heart, liver, kidney, spleen and lower extremities
iii Red and / or pale infarct Brain.

43. A. *Ref:* Harrison P–2092, HM P–439, COM P–156 & T.C.M.D.

Refer Q. 65.

- The Aschoff nodules or the Aschoff bodies are spheroidal or fusiform distinct tiny structures, 1-2 mm in size, occurring in the interstitium of the heart in RF and may be visible to naked eye.– HM
- RHD is the most common cause of disease in children in developing countries and is a major cause of mortality and morbidity in adults as well.
- Aschoff bodies are large cells with basophilic cytoplasm and a large vesicular nucleus, often multinucleated. They are characteristic of Aschoff's nodules.

Four

Respiratory System

QUESTIONS

1. **Bronze discolouration of oral mucosa is seen in:**
   A. Amalgam tattoo B. Neurilemoma
   C. Addison's disease D. Cushing disease

2. **The most frequent cause of non-inflammatory effusion in pleural cavity is:**
   A. Congestive cardiac failure
   B. Pulmonary embolism
   C. Nephrotic syndrome
   D. Bronchogenic carcinoma

3. **Clubbing is seen in all except:**
   A. Cancer of Lung B. Lung abscess
   C. Viral pneumonia D. Bronchiectasis

4. **Cigarette smoking causes all except:**
   A. Right ward shift
   B. Mobilization of FFA
   C. Mobilization of catecholamines
   D. None of the above

5. **Usually 'lobar pneumonia' is caused by:**
   A. Kleb pneumonia B. Strep. pyogenes
   C. H. influenza D. Pneumococci

6. **All of the following are features of primary tuberculosis except:**
   A. Weight loss and low grade fever
   B. Lower or mid lung zone pneumonitis

C. Enlarged hilar lymph node
D. Ghon complex

7. Lung abscess due to amoebiasis is because of:
A. Lymphatic spread
B. Hematogenous spread
C. Direct extension from liver
D. All of the above

8. Which test is most useful in the diagnosis of allergic rhinitis?
A. Peripheral blood smear
B. Immediate hypersensitivity skin test
C. Stained nasal smear for eosinophils
D. Measurement of serum IgE level

9. Bronchiectasis is:
A. Crackling sounds unaltered by coughing and are audible
B. Crackling sounds audible during inspiration
C. Chronic dilatation of a bronchus or bronchi, with a secondary infection that usually involves the lower portion of the lung
D. None of the above

10. All are true regarding pneumonia caused by Mycoplasma except:
A. It is highly contagious infection
B. It is diagnosed by presence of cold agglutinin antibodies
C. Erythromycin is used for treatment
D. It is difficult to culture

11. Decreased pleural fluid glucose is seen in all of the following except:
A. Empyema
B. Rheumatoid arthritis
C. Cirrhosis
D. Malignancy

12. All of the following are causes of decreased glucose in pleural effusion except:
A. Empyema
B. Cirrhosis

C. Squamous cell carcinoma
D. Rheumatoid arthritis

13. All of the following are seen in cerebellar lesions except:

A. Hypotonia B. Spontaneous tremors
C. Dysarthria D. Ataxia

14. The condition in which fluid is present in the pleural cavity is known as:

A. Hydrothorax B. Ascitis
C. Hydropericardium D. Hydroperitoneum

15. Most common cause of chronic bronchitis is:

A. Smoking
B. Silica dust inhalation
C. Asbestos dust inhalation
D. Coal dust inhalation

16. Which of the followings is most commonly implicated in silicosis?

A. Tridymite B. Quartz
C. Mica D. Talc

17. Which of the followings is not a type of extrinsic asthma?

A. Occupational asthma
B. Atopic asthma
C. Allergic bronchopulmonary aspergillosis
D. None of the above

18. Which of the followings is/are key players in allergic asthma?

A. Mast cells B. IgE
C. Eosinophils D. All of the above

19. "Blue bloaters" patients are suffering from:

A. Bronchial asthma B. Bronchitis
C. Atelectasis D. Emphysema

20. Which of the following conditions predispose to bronchiectasis:
   A. Cystic fibrosis
   B. Bronchial obstruction
   C. Kartagener's syndrome
   D. All of the above

21. Which of the following conditions is not associated with acute respiratory distress syndrome?
   A. Gastric aspiration
   B. Diffuse pulmonary infections
   C. Both of the above
   D. None of the above

22. Bronchopneumonia is most common in:
   A. Right middle lobe B. Lower lobes
   C. Both of the above D. None of the above

23. False negative result of tuberculin test occurs in:
   A. Hodgkin's disease B. Sarcoidosis
   C. Both of the above D. None of the above

24. Progressive pulmonary tuberculosis can lead to:
   A. Obliterative fibrous pleuritis
   B. Tuberculous empyema
   C. Pleural effusions
   D. All of the above

ANSWERS AND EXPLANATIONS WITH REFERENCES

1. **C.** *Ref:* Harrison P–2262, 2142, H M P–798, COM P–82 & SOP P–904
   - "Hyperpigmentation may be striking or absent. It commonly appears as a diffuse brown, tan, or BRONZE darkening parts such as the elbows or creases of the hand and of areas that normally are pigmented such as the areolae about the nipples. Bluish-black patches may appear on the mucous membrane."

- Harrison's; P–2142
- The original description of Addison's disease-"general languor and debility, feebleness of the heart's action, irritability of the stomach, and a peculiar change of the color of the skin"- dominant clinical features.
  Progressive chronic destruction of more than 90% of adrenal cortex on both sides results in an uncommon clinical condition called Addison's disease.–HM
- "Amalgam tattoo pigmentation appears as bluish gray or black macules on buccal mucosa, gingiva or palate."- COM P-82
- "Graphite tattoo appears as focal gray or black macules in school going children." –COM P-82
- "Due to an increased level of ACTH in the blood, the secretion of melanocyte stimulating hormone increases; which induces the deposition of melanin in the skin and mucous membrane."
- Shafer's; P–904

2. A.

- Congestive cardiac failure is the inability of the heart, working at normal or elevated filling pressure, to pump enough blood to supply the oxygen requirements of the body tissues. Congestive cardiac failure should never be considered a diagnosis. Rather, it is the syndrome resulting from many diseases that interfere with cardiac function.

3. C. *Ref:* Harrison P–1619 & COM P–162

- Pneumonia is an infection of the pulmonary parenchyma.
- Pneumonia or pneumonitis refers to inflammation of the lung parenchyma. The majority of cases of pneumonia are caused by virus.
- Bacteria, fungi and protozoa may also cause pneumonia.- COM
- The cause of clubbing of fingers and toes is not known. Digital clubbing is seen in advanced cases of bronchiec-

tasis and in some cases of lung abscess and lung cancer. It also may be a physical finding in patients with infiltrative lung disease (interstitial fibrosis). Digital clubbing is not seen in patients with chronic obstructive pulmonary disease (COPD).

4. C. *Ref:* Harrison P–1635 & HM P–497

- By 1964, the Advisory Committee to the Surgeon General of the United States had concluded that cigarette smoking was a major risk factor for mortality from chronic bronchitis and emphysema.
- The most important factor for high incidence of all forms of bronchogenic carcinoma is tobacco smoking. – HM
- Cigarette smokers are 60 present more likely to develop ASCAD than nonsmokers when other risk factors are controlled. Smoking increases carbon monoxide levels in the blood, which may in turn damage the coronary endothelium. Smoking also increases platelet adhesiveness and thus the likelihood of thrombotic coronary occlusion.

5. D. *Ref:* Harrison P–865, HM P–468 & TMD

- Pneumococci are identified in the clinical laboratory as catalase-negative, gram-positive cocci that grow in pairs or chains and cause ? hemolysis on blood agar. More than 98% of pneumococcal isolates are susceptible to ethylhydrocupreine (optochin), and virtually all pneumococcal colonies are dissolved by bile salts.
- More than 90% of all lobar pneumonias are caused by Streptococcus pnemoniae, a lancent-shaped diplococcus. Out of various type 3-S pneumoniae causes particularly virulent form of lobar pneumonia. – HM
- Pneumococci is an oval-shaped, encapsulated, non-spore-forming, gram positive organism occuring usually in pairs (diplococcus) and having lancet shaped ends.

6. A. *Ref:* HM P–153

- The infection of individual who has not been previously infected or immunized is called primary tuberculosis or Ghon's complex or childhood tuberculosis.– HM

- In reactivation tuberculosis weight loss and low grade fever occurs. The typical areas of involvement in reactivation tuberculosis are apical posterior segments of upper lobe and usually superior segments of lower lobe. Usually primary tuberculosis is asymptomatic.

7. C. *Ref:* Harrison P–1630, HM P–187

- Lung abscess is defined as pulmonary parenchymal necrosis and cavitation resulting from infection.
- Amoebiasis is caused by Enatamoeba histolytica named for its lytic action on tissues. It is the most important intestinal infection of man. The condition is particularly more common in tropical and subtropical areas with poor sanitation.– HM
- Lung abscess may be the result of a phylogenic pneumonia caused by pathogens such as S. aureus or S. pyogenes. More commonly, however, lung abscess occurs as a late stage in the evolution of untreated anaerobic or mixed flora (usually containing aerobes such as streptococci and anaerobes) pneumonia.

8. B. *Ref:* Harrison P–2068 & HM P–515

- Allergic rhinitis is characterized by sneezing; rhinorrhea; obstruction of the nasal passages; conjunctival, nasal, and pharyngeal itching; and lacrimation, all occurring in a temporal relationship to allergen exposure.
- Allergic rhinitis occurs due to sensitivity to allergens such as pollens. It is an IgE-mediated immune response consisting of an early acute response due to degranulaion mast cells, and a delayed prolonged response in which there is infiltration by leucocytes such as eosinophils, basophils, neutrophils and macrophages accompanied with oedema. –HM
- Most valuable tool for identifying the causative agent in allergic rhinitis is an accurately applied skin test.

9. C. *Ref:* HM P–484 & T.C.M.D.

- Bronchiectasis is defined as abnormal and irreversible dilation of the bronchi and bronchioles (greater than

2 mm in diameter) developing secondary to inflammatory weakening of the bronchial walls.– HM

- Dilatation may be in an isolated segment or spread throughout the bronchi. Acquired bronchiectasis usually occurs secondary to an obstruction or an infection such as bronchopneumonia, chronic bronchitis, tuberculosis, or whooping cough.

10. D.

- The causes of pneumonia are innumerable and include bacteria, viruses, fungi, and parasites. Identification of the specific cause of pneumonia, therefore, is necessary for effective treatment.

11. C. *Ref:* Harrison P–1971 & T.C.M.D.

- Cirrhosis is a condition that is defined histopathologically and has a variety of clinical manifestations and complications, some of which can be life-threatening.
- Cirrhosis is a chronic disease of the liver marked by formation of dense perilobular connective tissue, degenerative changes in the parenchymal cells, structural alteration of the cords of liver lobules, fatty and cellular infiltration, and sometimes development of areas of regeneration.

12. B. *Ref:* Harrison P–1971 & T.C.M.D.

- Cirrhosis is a condition that is defined histopathologically and has a variety of clinical manifestations and complications, some of which can be life-threatening.
- Cirrhosis is a chronic disease of the liver marked by formation of dense perilobular connective tissue, degenerative changes in the parenchymal cells, structural alteration of the cords of liver lobules, fatty and cellular infiltration, and sometimes development of areas of regeneration.

13. B.

- Spontaneous is without apparent cause said of disease processes or remissions.

14. A. *Ref:* Harrison P–266, HM P–505 & TMD

- A large pleural effusion, obscuring most of the lung, is known as a hepatic hydrothorax. The patient with diffuse abdominal swelling should be questioned about increased alcohol intake, a prior episode of jaundice or hematuria, or a change in bowel habits.
- Hydrothorax is non-inflammatory accumulation of serous fluid within the pleural cavities. Hydrothorax may be unilateral or bilateral depending upon the underlying cause. Occassionally, an effusion is limited to part of a pleural cavity by preexisting pleural adhesions. – HM
- Hydrothorax is a noninflammatory collection of fluid in the pleural cavity, causing dyspnea, an absence of vesicular breath sounds, murmur and flatness over the location of the fluid.

15. A. *Ref:* Harrison P–1635, HM P–477 & TMD

- By 1964, the Advisory Committee to the Surgeon General of the United states had concluded that cigarette smoking was a major risk factor for mortality from chronic bronchitis.
- The most commonly identified factor implicated in causation of chronic bronchitis and in emphysema is heavy smoking.
- Chronic bronchitis is marked by increased mucus secretion by the tracheobronchial tree. The productive cough is usually present for atleast 3 months of 2 consecutive years.

16. B. *Ref:* Harrison P–1614, HM P–490 & TMD

- In spite of the technical adequacy of existing protective equipment, free silica (SiO_2), or crystalline quartz, is still a major occupational hazard.
- Silicosis used to be called 'knife grinders' lung. Silicosis is caused by prolonged inhalation silicon dioxide, commonly called silica.– HM
- Quartz is a silicon dioxide, the principal ingredients of

sandstone (crystallized silica; rock crystal).When crystal is clear and colourless, it permits the passage of large amounts of ultraviolet radiations.

17. D. *Ref:* Harrison P–1596 & TMD

- A minority of asthmatic patients (approximately 10%) have negative skin test to common inhalant allergens and normal serum concentrations of IgE. These patients, with nonatopic or intrinsic asthma usually show later onset of disease (adult-onset asthma), commonly have concomitant nasal polyps, and may be aspirin-sensitive.
- Asthma is a disease caused by increased responsiveness of the tracheobronchial tree to various stimuli, which results in paroxysmal constriction of the bronchial airways. Asthma due to some environmental factors, usually allergic is called extrinsic asthma.

18. D. *Ref:* Harrison P–1596 & TMD

- Patients with asthma commonly suffer from other atopic disease, particularly allergic rhinitis which may be found in over 80% of asthmatic patients, and atopic dermatitis (eczema).
- Allergic asthma is a common form of asthma due to hypersensitivity to an allergen.

19. D. *Ref:* Harrison P–1640, COM P–160 & TMD

- Although traditional teaching is that patients with predominant emphysema, termed "pink puffers", are thin and noncyanotic at rest and have prominent use of accessory muscles, and patients with chronic bronchitis are more likely to be heavy and cyanotic ("blue bloaters"), current evidence demonstrates that most patients have elements of both bronchitis and emphysema and that the physical examination does not reliably differentiate the two entities.
- Emphysema refers to distension of the alveolar spaces due to presence of air. Clinical manifestation is breathlessness on exertion due to combined effect of reduction of alveolar surfaces for gas exchange and

collapse of smaller airways. Emphysema is usually the result of chronic bronchitis.– COM

- Emphysema is pathological distention of interstitial tissues by gas or air.

20. D. *Ref:* Harrison P–1629, HM P–484, 48, COM P–164 & TMD

- Bronchiectasis is an abnormal and permanent dilatation of bronchi.
- Several hereditary and congenital may result secondarily in diffuse bronmchiectasis:
  1. Cystic fibrosis, generlised defect of exocrine gland secretions, result in obstruction, infection and bronchietasis.
  2. Immotile cilia syndrome that includes Kartagener's syndrome (bronchietasis, situs inversus and sinusitis) is characterised by ultrastructural changes in the microtubules causing immotility of cilia of the respiratory tract epithelium, sperms and other cells. Males in this syndrome are often infertile.
  3. Atopic bronchial asthma patients have often positive family history of allergic diseases and may rarely develop diffuse bronchiectasis.– HM
- Cystic fibrosis or mucoviscidosis is an autosomal recessive inherited disorder of mucus producing exocrine glands. The disease prominently affects the lungs and pancreas. – COM
- Bronchiectasis is chronic dilatation of a bronchus or bronchi, with a secondary infection that usually involves the lower portion of the lung. Dilatation may be in an isolated segment or spread throughout the bronchi.

21. D. *Ref:* Harrison P–1680 & TMD

- Acute respiratory distress syndrome (ARDS) is a clinical syndrome of severe dyspnea of rapid onset, hypoxemia, and diffuse pulmonary infiltrates leading to respiratory failure.

- Acute respiratory distress syndrome is a clinical condition in which the patient's arterial oxygen concentration drops markedly with or without an increase in carbon dioxide concentration. In all cases, the diagnosis is made by comparing the previous "normal" baseline for the blood gas values with those in the acute situation.

22. **C.** *Ref:* HM P–471 & TMD

- Bronchopneumonia or lobular pneumonia is infection of the terminal bronchioles that extends into the surrounding alveoli resulting in patchy consolidation of the lung. –HM
- Bronchopneumonia is an inflammation of the alveoli, interstitial tissue, and bronchioles of the lungs due to infection by bacteria, viruses, or other pathogenic organisms, or to irritation by chemicals or other agents (e.g., oil, radiation, drugs).

23. **C.** *Ref:* HM P–369, 164, COM P–197 & TMD

- Hodgkin's disease (HD) primarily arises within the lymph nodes and involves the extranodal sites secondarily. This group comprises about 8% of all cases of lymphoid neoplasms. Sarcidosis is a systemic disease of unknown etiology. It is worldwide in distribution and effects adults from 20-40 years of age. – HM
- Hodgkin's disease is a malignant disease characterized by progressive involvement of lymphoid tissues.

  Sacoidosis is a granulomatous disease of unknown etiology, especially involving the lungs with resulting interstitial fibrosis. –COM
- Tuberculin test is a test to determine the presence of a tuberculosis infection based on a positive reaction of the subject to tuberculin. Tests do not reveal whether infection is active or inactive.

24. **D.** *Ref:* HM P–154, 155 & COM P–162

- The primary focus in the lung continues to grow and the gaseous material is disseminated through bronchi to the other parts of the opposite lung. This is called progressive primary tuberculosis. –HM

- Pulmonary tuberculosis is mostly transmitted from infected individual to others by inhalation of air droplets of sputum less than 8 micron in diameter. –COM
- Tuberculosis is the disease caused by infection with Mycobacterium tuberculosis, the tubercle bacillus, which can affect almost any tissue or organ of the body, the Progressive pulmonary tuberculosis is tuberculosis of the lungs.

Five

Renal Diseases

QUESTIONS

1. A 4 year child is having increased VMA urinary secretion could most probably have:
A. Neurolemmoma
B. Infancy neuroectodermal tumor
C. Hyperthyroidism
D. Multiple myeloma

2. Bence Jones protein found in the urine may be suggestive of:
A. Multiple myeloma
B. Hyperparathyroidism
C. Hodgkin's disease
D. Christian's syndrome

3. The important complication in diuretic phase of acute renal failure is:
A. Metabolic acidosis
B. Fulminant infection
C. Convulsions
D. Hypocalcaemia

4. In an elderly patient with anuria of sudden onset, the most likely diagnosis is:
A. Renal infarction
B. Urinary tract obstruction
C. Acute tubular necrosis
D. Acute cortical necrosis

5. Radiolucent renal stones are composed of:
A. Calcium
B. Cystine
C. Struvite
D. Urate (uric acid)

6. A patient with recurrent renal stones should be investigated for:

A. Proximal renal tubular acidosis
B. Hyperoxaluria
C. Increased ammonia levels
D. All the above

7. Increase in volume of both intravascular and interstitial fluids occurs in:

A. Nephrotic syndrome
B. Cirrhosis
C. Acute glomerulonephritis
D. All of the above

8. The hallmark of focal segmental glomerulosclerosis is:

A. Disruption of glomerular basement membrane
B. Disruption of endothelial cells of glomerular capillary
C. Disruption of visceral epithelial cells
D. None of the above

9. The nephritic syndrome is characterized by:

A. Hypotension
B. Uremia
C. Both of the above
D. None of the above

10. Which of the followings is absent in poststreptococcal glomerulonephritis ?

A. Granular deposits of IgG
B. Hypocomplementemia
C. Both of the above
D. None of the above

11. Presence of crescents in most of the glomeruli is characteristic feature of:

A. Lipid nephrosis
B. Rapidly progressive glomerulonephritis
C. Membranoproliferative glomerulonephritis
D. Acute proliferative glomerulonephritis

12. Berger's disease is:
   A. Type II rapidly progressive glomerulonephritis
   B. Thromboangiitis obliterans
   C. Type I rapidly progressive glomerulonephritis
   D. Immunoglobulin A nephropathy

13. Most common cause of acute renal failure is:
   A. Acute tubular necrosis
   B. Acute proliferative glomerulonephritis
   C. Acute pyelonephritis
   D. Malignant nephrosclerosis

14. Which of the followings is/are cause(s) of adrenal insufficiency ?
   A. Sarcoidosis
   B. Waterhouse-friderichsen syndrome
   C. Tuberculosis
   D. All of the above

ANSWERS AND EXPLANATIONS WITH REFERENCES

1. B. *Ref:* Harrison P–& SOP P–201
- "All the hematologic and blood chemistry values are within the normal range. The only finding in some but not all patients with MNTI (Melanotic neuroectodermal tumor of infancy) is an INCREASE IN THE URINARY LEVEL OF VMA, but shows no correlation with its clinical behaviour."
- The melanotic neuroectodermal tumor of infancy (MNTI) is a relatively uncommon osteolytic-pigmented neoplasm that primarily affects the jaws of newborn infants.
- Increased level of urinary VMA is also observed in pheochromocytoma and not in retinoblastoma, ganglioneuroblastoma, neuroblastoma; etc.

2. A. *Ref:* HM P–380, COM P–176 & SOP P–261, 262, Shafer's; P–261, 262; & Harrison's; P–251

- Multiple myeloma is a multifocal malignant proliferation of plasma cells derived from a single clone of cells. – HM
- Multiple myeloma is a malignant disease of plasma cells which are required for the humoral antibody response. These abnormal plasma cells produce myeloma protein instead of normal immunoglobulins. –COM
- "The Bence Jones protein in the urine is noted in 60-85 percent of multiple myeloma patients. This is an unusual protein which coagulates when the urine is heated to 40-600°C and then disappears when the urine is boiled. It reappears as urine is cooled." Shafer's; P-261, 262
- "Bence Jones proteins are light chains that undergo precipitation on heating and typically redissolve on further warming. 'Bence Jones protein' can be identified in the urine by its characteristics property of coagulation when heated to 500 °C but redissolving 700 °C."

3. D. *Ref:* Harrison P–1800 & HM P–836

- Hypocalcaemia may also result from the following:
  A. Due to renal dysfunction, there is decreased conversion of Vitamin D metabolic 25(OH) cholecalciferol to its active form 1,25 $(OH)_2$ cholcalciferol.
  B. Reduced intestinal absorption of calcium.–HM
- Inherited forms of hypochloremic metabolic alkalosis and hypokalemia without hypertension are due to genetic mutations of various ion transporters and channels of the thick ascending limb (TAL) of Henle's loop and distal convoluted tubule (DCT).
- Hypocalcemia is defined as serum calcium concentration of less than 8.5 mg/dl.

4. B. *Ref:* Harrison P–1820

- Acute inflections of the urinary tract fall into two general anatomic categories: lower tract infection (urethritis and cystitis) and upper tract infection (acute pyelonephritis, and intrarenal and perinephric abscesses).

- An obstruction in the urinary tract may occur at any point between the renal tubules and the urethra. Urinary obstruction may be acute or chronic, unilateral or bilateral, and partial or complete.

5. D. *Ref:* Harrison P–2444
- Uric acid is the final breakdown product of purine degradation in humans.
- Urate (uric acid), stones can not be detected by plain radiographs as they are radiolucent. They can be detected by IVP.

6. B. *Ref:* Harrison P–1755 & T.C.M.D.
- Hypovolemia or acidosis may further promote intra-tubular cast formation. Intratubular casts containing filtered immunoglobulin light chains and other proteins (including Tamm- Horsfdall protein produced by thick ascending limb cells) cause ARF in patients with multiple myeloma (myeloma cast nephropathy). Light chains are also directly toxic to tubule epithelial cells. Intra-tubular obstruction is an important cause of ARF in patients with severe hyperuricosuria or hyperoxaluria.
- Hyperoxaluria is in creased oxalic acid in the urine.

7. D. *Ref:* Harrison P–1790, 971, HM P–660, COM P–176 & TMD
- Nephrotic syndrome classically presents with heavy proteinuria, minimal hematuria, hypoalbuminemia, hypercholesterolemia, edema, and hypertension.
- Cirrhosis is a condition that is defined histopathologically and has a variety of clinical manifestations and complications, some of which can be life-threatening.
- Nephrotic syndrome is a constellation of features in different disease having varying pathogenesis; it is characterised by findings of massive proteinuria, hypoalbuminaemia, oedema, hyperlipidaemia, lipiduria, and hypercoagulability.

  Cirrhosis of the liver is one of the ten leading causes of death in the Western world.– HM

- In nephritic syndrome, damaged glomeruli lose large amount of serum protein that causes secondary hypogammaglobulinemia. Hpogammaglobulinemia leads to bacterial infections involving skin, lungs and oropharynx and may result in death in children with nephritic syndrome.– COM
- Cirrhosis is a chronic disease of the liver marked by formation of dense perilobular connective tissue, degenerative changes in the parencchymal cells, structural alteration of the cords of liver lobules, fatty and cellular infiltration and sometimes development of areas of regeneration. Nephritic syndrome is the end result of a variety of disease that damage the capillaries of the glomerulus. Acute glomerulonephritis, also known as acute nephritic syndrome, frequently follows infection, esp. those of the upper respiratory tract caused by particular strains of streptococci.

8. C. *Ref:* HM P–673

- Focal segmental glomerulosclerosis (FSGS) is a condition in which there is sclerosis and hyalinosis of some glomeruli and portions of their tuff (less than 50% in a tissue section), while the other glomeruli are normal by light microscopy i.e. involvement is focal and segmental. –HM
- Glomerulosclerosis is hyaline deposits or scarring within the renal glomeruli, a degenerative process occuring in association with renal arteriosclerosis or diabetes.

9. D.

- Nephritic syndrome is the inflammation of the kidney.

10. D. *Ref:* Harrison P–1782, 1783, HM P–665 & COM P–170

- Some glomerular diseases result from genetic mutations producing familiar disease. (1) Congenital nephritic syndrome from mutations in NPHS1 (nephrin) and NPHS2 (prodocin) affect the slit-pore membrane at birth, and TRPC6 cation channel mutations in adulthood produce focal segmental in genes encoding lamin A/C or PPARy cause a metabolic syndrome that can be associated with membranoproliferative glomerulonephritis (MPGN), which is sometime accompaniedby dence deposits and C 3 nephritic factor. (3) Alport's syndrome, from mutatins in the genes encoding for the α 3,α or α chains of type IV collagen, produces split-basement membranes with glomerulosclerosis.

- Acute post-streptococcal GN, though uncommon and sporadic in the western countries, is a common form of GN in developing countries, mostly affecting children between 2 to 14 years of age but 10% cases are seen in adults above 40 years of age. The onset of disease is generally sudden after 1-2 weeks of streptococcal infection, most frequently of the throat (e.g. streptococcal pharyngitis) and sometimes of the skin (e.g. streptococcal impetigo).

  There is usually hypocomplementaemia indicating involvement of complement in the glomerular deposits. –HM
- Glomerulonephritis is characterized by diffused inflammatory changes in glomeruli, that produce irreversible impairment of function. It may occur as acute glomerulonephritis which is of either streptococcal or non- streptococcal origin. – COM
- Glomerulonephritis is renal disease characterized by diffuse inflammatory changes in glomeruli that are not the acute response to infection of the kidneys.

Renal Diseases

11. B. *Ref:* HM P–667 & COM P–170
Refer Q. 187

- Rapidly progressive glomerulonephritis presents with an acute reduction in renal function resulting in acute renal failure in a few weeks or months. It is characterised by the formation of 'crescents' outside the glomerular capillaries. –HM
- Rapidly progressive glomerulonephritis is usually presenting insidiously, without preceding streptococcal

infection, with increasing renal failure leading to uremia within a few months; at autopsy the kidneys are normal in size, numerous glomerular capsular epithelial crescents are present, and antiglomerular basement membrane antibodies are frequently found.

12. **D.** *Ref:* HM P–674 & TMD

- IgA nephropathy is emerging as the most common form of glomerulopathy worldwide and its incidence has been rising. It is characterised by aggregates of IgA, deposited principally in the megnasium. –HM
- Immunoglobulin A is the principal immunoglobulin in exocrine secretions such as milk, respiratory and intestinal mucin saliva, and tears.

13. **A.** *Ref:* HM P–654 & TMD

- Intra-renal disease is characterised by disease of renal tissue itself. These include vascular disease of the arteries and arterioles within the kidney, disease of glomeruli, acute tubular necrosis due to ischaemia, or the effect of a nephrotoxin, acute tubulointerstitial nephritis and pyelonephritis. –HM
- Acute renal failure is acute failure of the kidney to perform its essential functions. It may be due to trauma; any condition that impairs the flow of blood to the kidneys; certain toxic substances such as mercury compounds, carbon tetrachloride, or ethylene glycol; bacteria toxins; glomerulonephriris; or acute obstruction of the urinary tract.

14. **D.** *Ref:* Harrison P–2264, HM P–798 & TMD

- All patients with adrenal insufficiency should receive specific hormone replacement. These patients require careful education about the disease.
- Causes of acute insufficiency are as under:
  1. Bilateral adrenalectomy e.g. in the treatment of cortical hyperfunction, hypertension and in selected cases of breast cancer.

2. Septicaemia e.g. in endotoxic shock and meningococcal infection producing grossly haemorrhagic and necrotic adrenal cortex termed adrenal apoplexy. The acute condition so produced is called Waterhouse-Fridertchsen's syndrome.
3. Rapid withdrawal of steroids.
4. Any form of acute stress in a case of chronic insufficiency i.e. in Addison's disease. –HM

- Adrenal insufficiency may be acute or chronic. The chronic form is called Addison's disease and is marked by anemia, sluggishness, weakness, weight loss, hypotension, sometimes hypoglycemia, nausea, vomiting, diarrhea, abnormal skin pigmentation and mental changes. The acute form is called adrenal crisis.

Six

Nervous System

QUESTIONS

1. **All of the following are characteristic features of petit mal seizures, except:**
   A. Short duration of seizures
   B. 3 Hz spike and wave pattern in EFG
   C. Onset after the age of 14 years
   D. Absence of motor activity during the seizures

2. **All of the following is true about CEREBRAL OEDEMA except:**
   A. Lymphatics and close apposition of cell processes of neurons and glia in the brain greatly increase the resorption of excess extracellular fluid.
   B. Interstitial edema occurs especially around the lateral ventricles.
   C. Herniation of brain occurs through foramen magnum.
   D. Allow fluid to escape from the intravascular compartment predominantly into the intercellular spaces of the brain.

3. **Calcification in the region of basal ganglion is least likely in:**
   A. Berry aneurysm
   B. Cysticerosis
   C. Idiopathic hypoparathyoidism
   D. Wilson's disease

4. **The drug of choice in complex partial seizures is:**
   A. Phenytoin B. Carbamazepine
   C. Sodium valproate D. Phenobarbitone

5. Autonomic neuropathy is seen in:
A. Diabetes mellitus B. Hyperglycemic coma
C. Epilepsy D. Hypertension

6. Multiple brain abscesses are characteristics of:
A. Hemorrhage B. Otitis media
C. Hematogenous D. Cyanotic heart disease

7. Wilson's disease is characterized by:
A. Low levels of ceruloplasmin
B. Low copper levels
C. High levels of ceruloplasmin
D. All of the above

8. In epileptic patient what has to be done first:
A. Maintain airway B. Give sedatives
C. Give cocktail regime D. Give phenytoin only

9. In classical migraine:
A. Attacks decrease with advancing age
B. Attacks can be aborted by early therapy
C. Aura may be absent
D. Diuresis is a recognized prodromal feature

10. Pyogenic meningitis is characterized by:
A. Increased protein, decreased glucose
B. Decreased protein, increased glucose
C. Decreased protein, decreased glucose
D. Increased protein, increased glucose

11. Most common site of bleeding in brain is:
A. Medulla
B. Putamen
C. Thalamus
D. Cerebral hemisphere

12. Most characteristic of Wilson's disease:
A. Decrease in serum ceruloplasmin
B. Increase in serum ceruloplasmin
C. Decrease is serum copper
D. None of the above

13. Defect in Broca's area causes:
   A. Defective expression of speech
   B. Defective fluency

14. Most common cause of cerebral infarction is:
   A. Embolism B. Venous thrombosis
   C. Hypertension D. Arterial thrombosis
   C. Defective understanding of speech
   D. Defective word formation

15. Trigeminal Neuralgia most often effects the:
   A. Left side nerve
   B. Both side nerves together
   C. Both side nerves equally
   D. Right side nerve

16. In case of cardiac arrest, brain activity is recorded by:
   A. Visual evoked response
   B. EEG
   C. CT scan
   D. Angiography

17. A young female who is conscious is suddenly unable to remember things. She is having:
   A. Conversion disorder
   B. Dissociative disorder
   C. Both of the above disorders
   D. Post-traumatic stress disorder

18. All of the followings are autosomal recessive except:
   A. Hemophilia
   B. Congenital adrenal hyperplasia
   C. Wilson's disease
   D. Cystic fibrosis

19. All of the followings are X linked transmissions except:
   A. Duchhenne's syndrome
   B. G6PD deficiency

C. Down's syndrome
D. Hemophilia

20. All of the following are seen in cerebellar lesions except:
A. Hypotonia
B. Spontaneous tremors
C. Dysarthria
D. Ataxia

21. Osteogenesis imperfecta is:
A. Sex-linked dominant disease
B. Autosomal dominant disease
C. Sex-linked recessive disease
D. Autosomal recessive disease

22. Which of the followings is most common chromosomal disorder?
A. Down syndrome
B. Turner syndrome
C. Fragile X syndrome
D. Klinefelter syndrome

23. Which of the following chromosomal features is/are seen in Kline filter syndrome case?
A. 46, XY
B. 47, XXY
C. 48, XXXY
D. All of the above

24. Peak sensitivity of embryo to teratogenesis occurs between:
A. Fourth and Fifth weeks of gestation
B. Second and Third weeks of gestation
C. Fifth and Sixth weeks of gestation
D. Third and Fourth weeks of gestation

25. Most common malignant eye tumor in childhood is:
A. Optoblastoma
B. Retinoblastoma
C. Neurofibromatosis
D. Teratoma

26. Flexner-wintersteiner rosettes are found in:
A. Retinoblastoma
B. Medullary adenoma
C. Neuroblastoma
D. Rhabdomyosarcoma

ANSWERS AND EXPLANATIONS WITH REFERENCES

1. C. *Ref:* Harrison P–2498, COM P–186 & T.C.M.D.

- A seizure is a paroxysmal event due to abnormal, excessive, hypersynchronous discharges from an aggregate of central nervous system (CNS) neurons.
- Petit Mal Seizure type of epileptic seizures occur in children and disappear during the second decade of life. The seizures lasts for seconds and occur without aura and little clonic or tonic phase. – COM
- Epilepsy is a recurrent paroxysmal disorder of cerebral function marked by sudden, brief attacks of altered consciousness, motor activity, or sensory phenomena. Convulsive seizures are the most common form of attack. Some but not all recurrent seizure patterns are not due to epilepsy.

2. A. *Ref:* Harrison's P–255, 2374 & HM P–101

- "Lymphatic and the close apposition of cell process of neurons and glia in the brain greatly IMPAIRS (i.e. decreases) the resorption of excess extra cellular fluid."
- Cerebral oedema or swelling of brain is the most threatening example of oedema.–HM
- "Because the cranial vault is subdivided by rigid dural folds (the falx and tentorium) a focal expansion of the brain causes it to be displaced in relation to these partitions. If the expansion is sufficiently severe, a herniation of the brain will occur." Robbin's P–1352

3. D. *Ref:* Harrison P–1981 & HM P–628

- Wilson's disease is an inherited disorder of copper homeostasis first described in 1912.
- Involvent of basal ganglia in the brain is seen in the form of toxic injury to neurons, in the cornea as greenish-brown deposits of copper in Descemet's membrane, and in the kidney as fatty and hydropic change.–HM

- Wilson's disease is an autosomal recessive disease characterized by excessive copper deposition, which, if untreated, may lead to fulminant hepatic failure. Copper also is deposited in the brain, kidney, and cornea, which causes Kayser-Fleischer rings. CNS disease may be prominent if the diagnosis is made in adulthood. Diagnosis is suggested by decreased serum ceruloplasmin levels and is confirmed by an increased hepatic copper concentration in a liver biopsy sample.

4. **B.** *Ref:* Harrison P–2507 & T.C.M.D.

- Carbamazepine (or a related drug, oxcarbazepine), phenytoin, lamotrigine and topiramate are currently the drugs of choice approved for the initial treatment of partial seizures, including those that secondarily generalize.
- Carbamazepine is a drug used for treatment of trigeminal neuralgia and temporal lobe epilepsy. It is used in psychiatry as a mood stabilizer in bipolar affective disorder. Trade names are Mezetol and Tegrital.

5. **A.** *Ref:* Harrison P–2289

- Individuals with long-standing type 1 or 2 DM may develop signs of autonomic dysfunction involving the cholinergic, noradrenergic, and peptidergic (peptides such as pancreatic polypeptide, substance P, etc.) systems.
- Diabetic neuropathy is common. Older patients with a relatively long history of diabetes and severe hyperglycemia have an increased incidence of the disease. Accumulation of sorbitol within Schwann cells, with subsequent cell damage, may play a causative role. Slowing of nerve conduction velocity occurs, with changes in Schwann cell function and eventual segmental demyelination.

6. **C.** *Ref:* Harrison P–2635 & HM P–201

- A brain abscess is a focal, suppurative infection within

the brain parenchyma, typically surrounded by a vascularized capsule.

- The sites where blood-borne metastasis commonly occurs are: the liver, lungs, brain, kidney and adrenals, all of which provide 'good soil' for the growth of 'good seeds' (seed-soil theory).–HM
- Hematogenous means pertaining to anything produced from, derived from, or transported by the blood.

7. A. *Ref:* Harrison P–1981 & HM P–628

- Wilson's disease is an inherited disorder of copper homeostasis first described in 1912.
  Refer Q 22
- Wilson's disease is an autosomal recessive disease characterized by excessive copper deposition, which, if untreated, may lead to fulminant hepatic failure. Copper also is deposited in the brain, kidney, and cornea, which causes Kayser-Fleischer rings. CNS disease may be prominent if the diagnosis is made in adulthood. Diagnosis is suggested by decreased serum ceruloplasmin levels and is confirmed by an increased hepatic copper concentration in a liver biopsy sample.

8. A. *Ref:* T.C.M.D.

- Epilepsy is a recurrent paroxysmal disorder of cerebral function marked by sudden, brief attacks of altered consciousness, motor activity, or sensory phenomena. Convulsive seizures are the most common form of attack. Some but not all recurrent seizure patterns are due not to epilepsy.

9. A. *Ref:* Harrison P–96, COM P–147 & T.C.M.D.

- Migraine, the second most common cause of headache, afflicts approximately 15% of women and 6% of men. It is usually an episodic headache that is associated with certain features such as sensitivity to light, sound, or movement; nausea and vomiting often accompany the headache. A useful description of migraine is a benign and recurring syndrome of headache associated with other symptoms of neurologic dysfunction in varying admixtures. Migraine can often be recognized by its activators, referred to as triggers.

- Migraine is a vascular disorder characterized by unilateral pain in the head. This pain usually begins before the age of 40 years and rarely begins in older individuals. Migraine headache can be divided into migraine with aura and migraine without aura. Aura is defined as subjective symptoms at the onset of or just before a migraine headache. – COM
- Migraine is a familial disorder marked by periodic, usually unilateral, pulsatile headaches that begin in childhood or early adult life and tend to recur with diminishing frequency in later life.

10. A. *Ref:* HM P–875 & T.C.M.D.

- Acute pyogenic or acute purulent meningitis is acute infection of the pia- arachnoid and of the CSF enclosed in the subarachnoid space. Since the subarachnoid space is continuous around the brain, spinal cord and the optic nerves, infection spreads immediately to whole of the cerebrospinal meanings as well as to the ventricles. –HM
- Meningitis is inflammation of the membranes of the spinal cord or brain.

11. B. *Ref:* T.C.M.D.

- Putamen is the darker outer layer of the lenticular nucleus.

12. A. *Ref:* Harrison P–1981& HM P–628

- Wilson's disease is an inherited disorder of copper homeostasis first described in 1912.
- Biochemical abnormalities in Wilson's disease include the following:
  1. Decreased serum ceruloplasmin (due to impaired synthesis of apoceruloplasmin in damaged liver and defective mobilisation of copper from hepatocellulr lysosomes).

2. Increased hepatic copper in liver biopsy (due to excessive accumulation of copper in the liver).
3. Increased urinary excretion of copper.
4. However, serum copper levels are of no diagnostic help and may vary from low-to-high depending upon the stage of disease.–HM

- Wilson's disease is an autosomal recessive disease characterized by excessive copper deposition, which, if untreated, may lead to fulminant hepatic failure. Copper also is deposited in the brain, kidney, and cornea, which causes Kayser-Fleischer rings. CNS disease may be prominent if the diagnosis is made in adulthood. Diagnosis is suggested by decreased serum ceruloplasmin levels and is confirmed by an increased hepatic copper concentration in a liver biopsy sample.

13. A. *Ref:* T.C.M.D.

- Broca's area is the area of the left hemisphere of the brain at the posterior end of the inferior frontal gyrus.

14. D.

- Infarction is sudden insufficiency of arterial or venous blood supply due to emboli, mechanical factors, or pressure that produces a macroscopic area of necrosis, any organ can be affected.

15. D. *Ref:* COM P–145

- Trigeminal neuralgia (TN) is characterized by severe, paroxysmal pain in one or more branches of trigeminal nerve. –COM
- In about 80 percent of the studies it has been observed that right side of the Trigeminal nerve is most often affected. The reason is unknown.

16. B. *Ref:* Harrison P–1708 & T.C.M.D.

- Cardiac arrest is abrupt cessation of cardiac pump function which may be reversible by a prompt intervention but will lead to death in its absence.
- Cardiovascular collapse is a sudden loss of effective blood flow due to cardiac and/or peripheral vascular factors

which may reverse spontaneously (e.g. neurocardiogenic syncope; vasovagal syncope) or only with interventions (e.g. cardiac arrest).
- Death is irreversible cessation of all biologic function.
- Cardiac arrest is sudden cessation of functional circulation.

17. B.

18. A. *Ref:* Harrison P–726 & HM P–335
- Hemophilia is an X-linked recessive hermorrhagic disease due to mutations in the F8 gene (hemophilia A or classic hemophilia) or F9 gene (hemophilia B). The disease affects 1 in 10,000 males worldwide, in all ethnic groups; hemophilia A represents 80%of all cases. Male subjects are clinically affected; women, who carry a single mutated gene, are generally asymptomatic. Family history of the disease is absent in approximately 30% of cases.
- Clinically, hemophilia A and hemophilia B are indistinguishable. The disease phenotype correlates with the residual activity of FVIII or FIX and can be classified as severe (< 1%), moderate (1-5%), or mild (6-30%).
- Classic hemophilia or hemophilia A is the second most common hereditary coagulation disorder next to von Willebrand's disease occurring due to deficiency or reduced activity of factor VIII (anti-hemophilic factor). – HM
- Hemophilia is the most common hereditary coagulopathy, accounting for 68 percent to 80 percent of such conditions.

19. C. *Ref:* HM P–258 &T.C.M.D.
- There is trisomy in about 95% cases of Down's syndrome due to nondisjunction during meiosis in one of the parents. Down's syndrome is the most common chromosomal disorder and is the commonest cause of mental retardation. The incidence of producing offspring

with Down's syndrome rises in mother over 35 years of age. – HM

- Transmission is transfer of anything, as a disease or hereditary characteristics.

20. B.

- Spontaneous is without apparent cause said of disease processes or remissions.

21. B. *Ref:* Harrison P–2463 & TMD

- Osteogenesis imperfecta is predominantly characterized by a generalized decrease in bone mass (osteopenia) and by brittle bones.
- Osteogenesis imperfecta is an inherited disorder of the connective tissue characterized by defective bone matrix with calcification occuring normally on whatever matrix is present.

22. A. *Ref:* TMD

- Down syndrome is a variety of congenital moderate-to-severe mental retardation.

23. D. *Ref:* TMD

- Kline filter syndrome is congenital endocrine condition of primary testicular failure usually not evident before puberty. The classic form is associated with presence of an extra X-chromosome.

24. A. *Ref:* TMD

- Teratogenesis is causing abnormal development of the embryo.

25. B. *Ref:* TMD

- Retinoblastoma is a malignant glioma of the retina, usually unilateral, that occurs in young children and usually is hereditary.

26. A. *Ref:* TMD

- Retinoblastoma is the initial diagnostic finding is usually a yellow or white light reflex seen at the pupil (cat's eye reflex).

Seven

Endocrine and Metabolic Disorders

QUESTIONS

1. **Which amongst the following is used in the treatment of diabetes insipidus?**
   A. Thiazide
   B. Carbonic anhydrase inhibitors
   C. Spironolactone
   D. Lithium carbonate

2. **The following conditions are known to occur more commonly in females, except:**
   A. Rheumatoid arthritis
   B. Thyrotoxicosis
   C. Ankylosing spondylitis
   D. Systemic lupus erythematosis

3. **About thyrotoxicosis all are true except:**
   A. Non ejection systolic click
   B. Ejection systolic click
   C. Early diastolic click
   D. Tremors

4. **Tertiary hyperparathyroidism is characterized by:**
   A. Autonomous chief cell hyperplasia
   B. Primary and secondary exaggerated
   C. Thyroid surgery complication
   D. Pituitary hyperplasia

5. **In diabetes mellitus, which nerve is involve:**
   A. III B. VI
   C. IV D. V

6. Drug of choice for acute gout is:
A. Sulfinpyrazone B. Indomethacin
C. Probenicid D. Allopurinol

7. Autoimmune arthritis is seen in:
A. Rheumatoid arthritis
B. Psoriatic arthritis
C. Osteoarthritis
D. Suppurative

8. In rheumatoid arthritis all of the following are seen except:
A. Symmetric joint involvement
B. Low back pain
C. Involvement of small joints
D. Early morning stiffness

9. A diabetic was suffering from orbital mucoromycosis. The treatment to be given to him should include:
A. Amphotericin B
B. Ltraconazole
C. Fluconazole
D. Ketoconazole

10. Diabetes mellitus is a chronic disorder of:
A. Protein metabolism
B. Fat metabolism
C. Carbohydrate metabolism
D. All of the above

11. Long-standing diabetes mellitus causes (s):
A. Microangiopathy B. Nephropathy
C. Retinopathy D. All of the above

12. Second most common cause of death from diabetes mellitus is:
A. Diabetic nephropathy
B. Myocardial infarction
C. Autonomic neuropathy
D. Diabetic microangiopathy

13. Deficiency of insulin affect(s):

A. Fat metabolism B. Glucose metabolism
C. Protein metabolism D. All of the above

14. Which of the followings is also known as Wermer's syndrome?

A. Multiple endocrine neoplasia IIa
B. Multiple endocrine neoplasia I
C. Multiple endocrine neoplasia IIb
D. Multiple endocrine neoplasia

15. Cushing's syndrome is caused by:

A. Hypercortisolism
B. Hyperadrenalism
C. Acute adrenal insufficiency
D. Chronic adrenal insufficiency

16. Which of the followings does not cause osteoporosis?

A. Hypoparathyroidism B. Hyperparathyroidism
C. Hypothyroidism D. Hyperthyroidism

17. The fading of cellular chromatin is:

A. Cytolysis B. Pyknosis
C. Karyolysis D. Karyorrhexis

18. Osteomalacia is associated with:

A. Increase in osteoid maturation time
B. Decrease in osteoid surface
C. Decrease in osteoid volume
D. Increase in mineral apposition rate

ANSWERS AND EXPLANATIONS WITH REFERENCES

1. A. *Ref:* HM P–795 & COM P–190

- The main features of diabetes insipidus are excretion of a very large volume of dilute urine of low specific gravity (below 1.010), polyuria and polydipsia. –HM
- The main aim of the treatment of diabetes insipidus to achieve normal or close to normal blood sugar and

prevention of diabetic complications. Diet, exercise, weight control and medications are the mainstays of management. – COM

- Thiazide any of a group of benzo-thiadiazine sulfonamide derivatives, typified by chlorothiazide, that act as diuretics by inhibiting the resorption of sodium in the proximal renal tubule and stimulating chloride excretion, with resultant increase in excretion of water.

2. **C.** *Ref:* Harrison P–2109 & HM P–853
- Ankylosing spondylitis (AS) is an inflammatory disorder of unknown cause that primarily affects the axial skeleton; peripheral joints and extraarticular structures are also frequently involved.
- Ankylosing spondylitis or rheumatoid spondylitis is rheumatoid involvement of the spine, particularly sacroiliac joints, in young male patients. –HM
- However, women tend to have asymptomatic or very mild disease with more peripheral joint manifestations.

3. **C.** *Ref:* Harrison P- 2233 & HM P–802
- Thyrotoxicosis is defined as the state of thyroid hormone excess and is not synonymous with hyperthyroidism. Hyperthyroidism, also called thyrotoxicosis, is a hypermetabolic clinical and biochemical state caused by excess production of thyroid hormones. – HM
- Thyrotoxicosis is the state produced by excessive quantities of endogenous or exogenous thyroid hormone. (Thyro- + G. toxikon, poison, + -osis, condition).

4. **A.** *Ref:* HM P– 817
- Tertiary hyperparathyroidism is a complication of secondary hyperparathyroidism in which the hyperfunction persists in spite of removal of the cause of secondary hyperplasia. Possibly, a hyperplastic nodule in the parathyroid gland develops which becomes partially autonomous and continues to secrete

large quantities of parathyroid hormone without regard to the needs of the body.–HM

- Elevation of the serum calcium level is the hallmark of primary hyperparathyroidism.
- Emergency treatment of hypercalcemia is necessary if the calcium level rises to very high levels (higher than 13 to 15 mg/dl) before the adenoma can be removed or if surgical treatment is refused or is unsuccessful.

5. A. *Ref:* HM P–824

It is known that in both type 1 and 2 DM, severity and chronicity of hyperglycaemia forms the main pathogenetic mechanism for 'microvascular complications' (e.g. retinopathy, nephropathy, neuropathy); therefore control of blood glucose level constitutes the mainstay of treatment for minimizing development of these complications. –HM

- Diabetic neuropathy is common. Older patients with a relatively long history of diabetes and severe hyperglycemia have an increased incidence of the disease. Accumulation of sorbitol within Schwann cells, with subsequent cell damage, may play a causative role. Slowing of nerve conduction velocity occurs, with changes in Schwann cell function and eventual segmental demyelination.

6. B. *Ref:* HM P–853 & TMD

- Gout is a disorder of purine metabolism manifested by the following features, occurring singly or in combination:
  1. Increased serum uric acid concentration (hyperuricaemia).
  2. Recurrent attacks of characterstic type of acute arthritis in which crystals of monosodium urate monohydrate may be demonstrable in the leucocytes present in the synovial fluid.
  3. Aggregated deposits of monosodium urate monohydrate (tophi) in and around the joints of the extremities.

4. Renal disease
5. Uric acid nephrolithiasis. – HM

- Indomethacin is the prototypical drug of this category and the one usually selected when the diagnosis of gout is secure and contraindications to the drug are not present.
- Indomethacin is an anti-inflammatory, analgesic and antipyretic drug. Its primary use is in rheumatoid arthritis, ankylosing, spondilitis etc.

7. A. *Ref:* Harrison P–2083, HM P–851 & COM P–179

- Rheumatoid arthritis (RA) is a chronic multisystem disease of unknown cause.
- Rheumatoid arthritis (RA) is a chronic multisystem disease of unknown cause. Though the most prominent manifestation of RA is inflammatory arthritis of the peripheral joints, usually with a symmetrical distribution, its systemic manifestations include haematologic, pulmonary, neurological and cardiovascular abnormalities. – HM
- Rheumatoid arthritis (RA) is characterized by inflammation of the synovial membrane. Females are about 3 times more affected usually between the age group of 35 to 50 years. Weakness and fatigue followed by stiffness of joints occurs. –COM
- Rheumatoid arthritis initiates a nonspecific immune response. The joint lesion in rheumatoid arthritis begins as an inflammatory lesion in the synovial membrane that can progress to a proliferative one (the pannus), which can deform by destroying adjacent cartilage and bone.

8. B. *Ref:* Harrison P–2083, HM P–851,1932 & COM P–140

- Rheumatoid arthritis (RA) is a chronic multisystem disease of unknown cause.
  Refer Q. 87
- Rheumatoid arthritis usually affects both the joints. Pain

and restriction of mouth opening are the most common symptoms. –COM

- The metacarpophalangeal and proximal interphalangeal joints of the hands, wrists, knees, and the metatarsophalangeal and proximal interphalangeal joints of the feet are the most common joints involved initially. Typically, patients have polyarticular, bilaterally symmetrical disease.

9. A. *Ref:* T.C.M.D.

- Amphotericin B is an antibiotic agent obtained from a strain of Streptomyces nodosus. It is used in treatment of deep-seated mycotic infections. The drug usually is administered parenterally. Trade name is Fungizone.

10. D. *Ref:* Harrison P–2275, HM P–818 & TMD

- Diabetes mellitus (DM) refers to group of common metabolicdisorders that share the phenotype of hyperglycemia.
- As per the WHO, diabetes mellitus (DM) is defined as a heterogeneous metabolic disorder characterised by common feature of chronic hyperglycaemia with disturbance of carbohydrate, fat and protein metabolism. –HM

– Diabetes mellitus is a group of forms of diabetes mellitus that occur predominantly in adults. The insulin produced is sufficient to prevent ketoacidosis but insufficient to meet the total needs of the body.

11. D. *Ref:* Harrison P–2275, HM P–826, COM P–189, 190 & TMD

- Diabetes mellitus (DM) refers to group of common metabolic disorders that share the phenotype of hyperglycemia.
- Diabetic microangiopathy: Microangiopathy of diabetes is characterised by basement membrane thickening of small blood vessels and capillaries of different organs and tissues such as the skin, skeletal muscle, eye and kidney.

- Diabetic nephropathy: Renal involvement is a common complication and a leading cause of death in diabetes.
- Diabetic neuropathy: Diabetic neuropathy may affect all parts of the nervous system but symmetric peripheral neuropathy is most characteristic. –HM
- Diabetic retinopathy may be progressive color blindness to total blindness due to involvement of retina in diabetes.

  Diabetic nephropathy is a major cause of mortality in diabetics and affects 50% of the patients with Type I diabetes. –COM
- Diabetes mellitus is a form of diabetes in nonobese patients can usually be controlled by diet and oral hypoglycemic agents, such as sulfonylurea drugs or metformin, a nonsulfonyl urea drug. In diabetes mellitus occasionally insulin therapy is required, in obese patients the condition can be controlled by avoidance of overfeeding.

12. A. *Ref:* Harrison P–2303, HM P–826 & TMD

- As with any chronic, debilitating disease, the individual with DM faces a series of challenges that affect all aspects of daily life. Emotional stress may provoke a change in behavior so that individuals no longer adhere to a dietary, exercise or therapeutic regimen.
- Renal involvement is a common complication and a leading cause of death in diabetes. Four types of lesions are described in diabetic nephropathy:
  1. Diabetic glomerulosclerosis
  2. Vascular lesions
  3. Diabetic pyelonephritis and necrotizing renal papillitis
  4. Tubular lesions or Armanni-Ebstein lesion. –HM
- Nephropathy is a disease of kidney. This term includes inflammatory (nephritis), degenerative (nephrosis), and sclerotic (artrtioscleriotic) lesion of the kidney.

13. D. *Ref:* HM P–819 & TMD

- The major stimulus for both synthesis and release of insulin is glucose.

- Glucose is the key regulator of insulin secretion from β-cells by a series. –HM
- Insulin is a hormone secreted by the beta cells of the islets of Langerhans of the pancreas.

14. **B.** *Ref:* HM P–829

- Multiple endocrine neoplasia type I syndrome (Wermer's syndrome) includes adenomas of the parathyroid glands, pancreatic islets and pituitary. The syndrome is inherited as an autosomal dominant trait. – HM
- Wermer's syndrome is an autosomal-dominant predisposition to tumors of parathyroid glands, anterior piturity, endocrine pancreas, and less commonly, other organs.

15. **A.** *Ref:* Harrison P–2254 & HM P–797

- Cushing described a syndrome characterized by turncal obesity, hypertension, fatigability and weakness, amenorrhea, hirsutism, purplish abdominal striae, edema, glucosuria, osteoporosis, and a basophilic tumor of the pituitary.
- Cushing's Syndrome (Chronic Hypercortisolism) is caused by excessive production of cortisol of whatever cause. The full clinical expression of the syndrome, however, includes contribution of the secondary derangements. –HM
- Cushing syndrome is a disorder resulting from increased adrenocortical secretion of cortisol.

16. **A.** *Ref:* Harrison P–2392 & HM P–835

- Hereditary hypoparathyroidism can occur as an isolated entity without other endocrine or dermatologic manifestations (idiopathic hypoparthyroidism).
- Osteoporosis may be difficult to distinguish radiologically from other osteoporosis such as osteomalacia, osteogensis imperfecta, osteitis fibrosa of hyperparathyroidism, renal osteodystrophy and multiple myeloma. –HM

- Hypoparathyroidism is a condition due to diminution or absence of the secretion of parathyroid harmones, with low serum calcium and tetany, and sometimes with increased bone density.

17. **C.** *Ref*-: HM P–30

- The nucleproteins are damaged by the activated lysosomal enzymes such as proteases and endonucleases. Irreversible damage to the nucleus can be in three forms:
  1. Pyknosis: Condensation and clumping of nucleus which becomes dark basophilic.
  2. Karyorrhexis: Nuclear fragmentation into small bits dispersed in the cytoplasm.
  3. Karylysis: Dissolution of the nucleus. –HM
- Pyknosis: Condensation of nuclear chromatin
- Karyolysis: Dissolution or fading of nuclear chromatin
- Cytolysis: Separation or division of cytoplasm.
- Karyorrhexis: Fragmentation of chromatin material into many granular clumps.

18. **A.** *Ref*: Harrison P–2375 & HM P–250

- The hypocalcemia and hypophosphatemia that accompany vitamin D deficiency result in impaired mineralization of bone matrix proteins, a condition known as osteomalacia.
- Osteomalacia is the adult counterpart of rickets in which there is failure of minerlisation of the osteoid matrix. –HM

Eight

Infections

QUESTIONS

1. **Following dental manipulation the most common organism carrying infective endocarditis is:**
   A. Staph. aureus
   B. Group A streptococci
   C. Gram-negative rod
   D. Streptococcus viridians

2. **In anemia of chronic disorders following increase/s:**
   A. Serum Fe B. Ferritin
   C. None of the above D. Both of the above

3. **All the following organisms can cause infectious bloody diarrhea except:**
   A. Entamoeba histolytica
   B. Giardia lambia
   C. Shigella
   D. Campylobacter

4. **Drug not used in pseudomonas infection is:**
   A. Imipenam B. Ceftazidime
   C. Pefloxacin D. Azithromycin

5. **The mother is HIV positive. The earliest time when the infection can be checked in the fetus is:**
   A. 8 weeks B. 22 weeks
   C. 15 weeks D. 28 weeks

6. **The treatment of choice for intestinal and extraintestinal amebiasis is:**
   A. Diloxanide furoate B. Tetracycline
   C. Metronidazole D. Chloroquin

7. A patient with a dog bite on the face should be treated with:

A. Antirabies vaccine and immunoglobin are to be administered at the same time

B. Initially vaccine is given followed later by immunoglobulins

C. Local treatment and vaccine only

D. Antirabies vaccine need only be given

8. In a 30 years old male patient the lymph nodes enlargement show necrosis with poor granuloma formation with plenty of acid fast bacilli. He may be suffering from:

A. Sarcoidosis

B. Mycobacteria bovis infection

C. Tuberculosis in an immuno-competent patient

D. HIV with tuberculosis

9. Infants with DiGeorge's syndrome are extremely vulnerable to:

A. Fungal infection B. Viral infection

C. Protozoal infection D. All of the above

10. Which fibril protein is mainly present in familial Mediterranean fever?

A. 2 microglobulin B. Amyloid light chain

C. Procalcitonin D. Amyloid associated

11. Diarrhea due to exudative diseases occurs because of:

A. Salmonella B. Shigella

C. Campylobacter D. All of the above

12. Which of the followings is not included in Hutchinson's triad?

A. Deafness

B. Notched central incisors

C. Fused teeth

D. Interstitial keratitis

ANSWERS AND EXPLANATIONS WITH REFERENCES

1. **D.** *Ref:* Harrison P–1004, HM P0–180 & TMD

- Endocarditis due to anaerobes is uncommon. However, anaerobic streptococci, which are often classified incorrectly, are responsible for this disease more frequently than is generally appreciated.
- Untypable?-haemolytic strepcocci such as Streptococcus viridans constitute the normal flora of the mouth and may cause bacterial endocarditis.–HM
- Endocarditis is an inflammation of the lining membrane of the heart. It is usually confined to covering of a valve and some times to the lining membrane of the chambers.

2. **C.** *Ref:* Harrison P–1167, COM P–176 & T.C.M.D.

- The CD4+T cell count is the laboratory text generally accepted as the best indicator of the immediate state of immunologic competence of the patient with HIV infection.
- Acquired Immunodeficiency Syndrome (AIDS)
  Immunopathogenesis
  A. Human immunodeficiency virus has ability to suppress cell-mediated immunity by infecting T4 cells, the helper lymphocytes. These lymphocytes contain CD4 surface
  molecule which bind the virus to the cell.
  B. HIV decreases T4 lymphocyte count below 200 mm^3, at which the patient becomes susceptible to infections and tumors.
  C. Infection with HIV causes abnormalities of monocytes and natural killer cells (macrophages). – COM
- Helper T. cell is a type of T lymphocyte needed for the production of antibodies against certain antigens.

3. **B.** *Ref:* Harrison P–1311

- Giardia lambia (also known as G.intestinalis) is a cosmopolitan protozoal parasite that inhabits the small intestines of humans and other mammals.

- Giardia lambia is not an invasive parasite like the rest hence does not cause bloody diarrhea.

4. D. *Ref:* Harrison P–1037

- Azithromycin is a macrolide that belongs to the family of azalides.
- Pseudomonas is a genus of motile, polar-flag-ellate, non-spore-forming, strictly aerobic bacteria (family Pseudomondaceae) containing straight or curved, but not helical Gram-negative rods that occur singly.

5. A *Ref:* TMD

- Babies born to HIV-positive mothers are tested for HIV-antibodies at birth and at 1,3 and 6 months.

6. C.

- Metronidazole has broad spectrum cidal activity against protozoa, including Giardia Lamblia in addition to the above two. Many anaerobic bacteria, such as Bact. fragilis, Fusobacterium, Clostridium perfringens, anaerobic Streptococci and the helminth Dracunculus medinensis are sensitive. It does not affect aerobic bacteria. Clinically significant resistance has not developed among the parasites for which it is used.

7. A.

- Rabies vaccine was introduced by Pasteur as a method of treatment for the bite of a rabid animal.

8. D. *Ref:* Harrison P–10, HM P–72, COM P–129 & T.C.M.D.

- Symptoms pertaining to lungs develop in about 50-75% of cases and are a major cause of death in HIV/AIDS. These features are largely due to opportunistic infections causing pneumonia, e.g. with Pneumocystis carinii, M. tuberculosis, CMV, Histoplasma, and Staphylococci. Lung abscess too may develop. Other pulmonary manifestations include adult respiratory distress syndrome and secondary tumours (e.g. Kaposi's sarcoma, lymphoma). –HM

- Tuberculosis is chronic bacterial infection which leads to the formation of granulomas in the infected tissues. Usually lungs are involved. Other tissues like lymph nodes, salivary glands may be involved. TB patients may feel xerostomia with or without swelling of salivary glands. The affected salivary gland may have granuloma or/and cyst. -COM
- A substantial proportion of the resurgence of TB registered in southern Africa may be attributed to HIV co-infection. Even before the advent of HIV, however, it was estimated that fewer than half of all cases of TB in developing countries were ever diagnosed, much less treated.
- Tuberculosis is most commonly seen in homeless people, refugees from Asia, those in prisons and long-term psychiatric facilities, the elderly, particularly those in residential facilities, and people infected with HIV.

9. **D.** *Ref:* Harrison P–2057, COM P–223 &TMD

- This classic example of isolated T cell deficiency results from maldevelopment of thymic epithelial elements derived from the third and fourth pharyngeal pouches. The gene defect has been mapped to chromosomal position 22q11 in most patients with the diGeorge syndrome, and to 10p in others
- Immunosuppressed patients are also susceptible to fungal infections. Fungal infections include candidiasis, cryptococcosis, mucormycosis, blastomycosis and asperillosis.

  Viral infections are common complication in immunosuppressed patients. – COM
- An infection produced by single-celled organism, such as amebic dysentery, sleeping sickness, and malaria is called Di-George's syndrome.

10. **D.** *Ref:* TMD

- Familial Mediterranean fever is a disease originally common in people of the middle east, but now it is seen in various parts of the world.

11. D. *Ref:* Harrison 247 & TMD

- Diarrhea is loosely defined as passage of abnormally liquid or unformed stools at an increased frequency.
- Diarrhea is a state in which an individual experiences a change in normal bowel habits characterized by the frequent passage of loose, fluids and uniform stools.

12. C. *Ref:* HM P–163

- The main major morphologic of congenital syphilis features as under:
  1. Saddle-shaped nose deformity due to destruction of bridge of the nose.
  2. The characteristic 'Hutchinson's teeth' which are small, widely spaced, peg-shaped permanent teeth.– HM
- Hutchinson's triad is parenchymatous keratitis, labyrinthine disease, and Hutchinson teeth, significant of congenital syphilis.

Nine

Medical Emergencies in Dental Practices

QUESTIONS

1. **Treatment of Tetralogy of Fallot include all of the following except:**
   A. Give morphine B. Give O2s
   C. Propanolo D. Shunt operation
2. **All of the following are used in the treatment of hypertensive emergencies except:**
   A. Nifedipine B. Sodium Nitropruside
   C. Prazosin D. Nitroglycerin
3. **What is the color of skin in case of acute poisoning of carbon monoxide?**
   A. Dull pink B. Red color
   C. Cherry red D. Coral pink

ANSWERS AND EXPLANATIONS WITH REFERENCES

1.C. *Ref:* HM P–425 & COM P–157

- Tetralogy of Fallot is the most common cyanotic congenital heart disease, found in about 10% of children with anomalies of the heart. –HM
- Tetralogy of Fallot is a congenital heart defect that includes ventricular hypertrophy. Oral manifestations are cyanosis of the oral mucosa, fissured and edematous tongue, marginal gingivitis and delayed eruption of deciduous and permanent teeth. –COM

- Tetralogy means a group or series of fourt of fallot is a complex of congenital heart defects consisting of pulmonic stenosis, interventricular septal defect, hypertrophy of right ventricle, and dextroposition of the aorta.

2. C. *Ref:* T.C.M.D.

- Prazosin hydrochloride is a drug used in treating hypertension. It acts as an alpha-adrenergic receptor blocker.

3. A. *Ref:* TMD

- Retinoblastoma is the initial diagnostic finding is usually a yellow or white light reflex seen at the pupil (cat's eye reflex).

Ten

Critical Care

QUESTIONS

1. Which of the following is not the cause of severe adverse drug effects?

A. Diabetes B. Death

C. Prolong hospital stay D. Immobilization

ANSWERS AND EXPLANATIONS WITH REFERENCES

1. C. *Ref:* Harrison's P- 13-24

- "Prolong Hospital stay is the cause of 'minor' and 'moderate' adverse effects not severe adverse effects."

Adverse Drug Effects

Minor | Moderate | Severe | Lethal

Prolong hospital stay

A. Minor adverse effects:

i. No therapy

ii. Antidote

iii. Prolongation of hospitalization required.

B. Moderate adverse effects:
   i. Requires change in drug therapy.
   ii. Specific treatment.
   iii. Prolongs hospital stay.

C. Severe adverse effects:
   i. Causes permanent damage (that means immobilization can occur due to permanent damage of nerve).
   ii. Potentially life threatening.
   iii. Requires intensive medical treatment.

D. Lethal adverse effects:
   i. Directly or indirectly contributes to the death of the patient.

Eleven

Anaphylaxis and Drug Allergy

QUESTIONS

1. A patient with anaphylactic shock which one should be administered first:

A. Corticosteroids B. Oxygen
C. Antihistaminics D. Adrenaline

ANSWERS AND EXPLANATIONS WITH REFERENCES

1. D.

- Anaphylactic shock causes death due to laryngeal oedema and bronochospasm which is reversed only by adrenaline. Though all of the above have to be administered, but during emergency most effective is adrenaline.

Twelve

Nutrition

QUESTIONS

1. Niacin deficiency leads to the development of:

A. Diarrhea B. Peripheral neuritis
C. Cheilosis D. Photophobia

2. Pseudofracture is classically seen in:

A. Hypoparathyroidism
B. Pseudohypoparathyroidism
C. Osteoporasis
D. Osteomalacia

3. The deficiency of which of the following vitamins can be assessed by measuring and following the transketolase enzyme in the red blood cell:

A. Folic acid B. Thiamine
C. Niacin D. Vitamin B2

4. Rickets like features occurs in all except:

A. Renal tudular acidosis
B. Hyperparathyroidism
C. Metaphyseal osteoporosis
D. Long-term intake of anticonvulsants

5. Which of the following infant factors is associated with sudden infant death syndrome (SIDS)?

A. Low birth weight B. Male sex
C. First sibling D. None of the above

6. Most active form of vitamin D is formed in:

A. Skin B. Lung
C. Kidney D. Liver

7. Which of the followings is/are a feature of rickets?
A. Squared appearance of head
B. Rachitic rosary
C. Pigeon chest deformity
D. All of the above

8. Wernicke encephalopathy is associated with:
A. Cyanocobalamin B. Thiamine
C. Biotin D. Folate

9. Vitamin C is needed for activation of :
A. Lysyl hydroxylase B. Prolyl hydroxylase
C. Both of the above D. None of the above

10. Acrodermatitis enteropathica is associated with deficiency of :
A. Nickel B. Zinc
C. Iron D. Copper

11. What is the value of normal Body Mass Index (BMI)?
A. 35 kg/M2 B. 15 kg/M2
C. 20 kg/M2 D. 25 kg/M2

ANSWERS AND EXPLANATIONS WITH REFERENCES

1. **A.** *Ref:* Harrison P–247 & HM P–253
   - Diarrhea is loosely defined as passage of abnormally liquid or unformed stools at an increased frequency Lesions similar to those seen in skin may develop in mucous membrane of the alimentary tract-resulting in glossitis, lesions in the mouth, oesophagus, stomach and colon and cause diarrhea, nausea, vomiting and burning sensation.–HM
   - Diarrhea is defined as an increase in stool frequency and volume. The stool usually is liquid, and 24 hour output exceeds 250 g. The patient may experience lower abdominal crampy pain and fecal urgency.

2. D. *Ref:* Harrison P–2375 & HM P–250

- The hypocalcemia and hyphosphatemia that accompany vitamin D deficiency result in impaired mineralization of bone matrix proteins, a condition known as osteomalacia.
- Osteomalacia is the adult counterpart of rickets in which there is failure of mineralization of the osteoid matrix. –HM
- Osteomalacia is a disease characterized by a gradual softening and bending of the bones with varying severity of pain.

3. B. *Ref:* Harrison P–441 &T.C.M.D.

- Thiamine was the first B vitamin to be identified and is therefore also referred to as Vitamin B1.
- Moderate deficiency of thiamine results in impaired functioning of nervous, circulatory, digestive, and endocrine systems. Neurasthenia, neurological disorders, and cardiac and gastrointestinal symptoms may result. Loss of appetite, fatigue, muscle tenderness, and increased irritability are symptoms. Severe prolonged deficiency results in beriberi.

4. C. *Ref:* Harrison P–2375 & HM P–249

- In children, prior to epiphyseal fusion, vitamin D deficiency results in growth retardation associated with an expansion of the growth plate known as Rickets.
- The primary defects in rickets are:
  A. interference with mineralization of bone; and
  B. deranged endochondral and intramembranous bone growth.– HM
- Rickets is a disease due to vitamin D deficiency and characterized by overproduction and deficient calcification of osteoid tissue, with associated skeletal deformities, disturbances in growth, hypocalcemia, and sometimes tetany; usually accompanied by irritability, listlessness, and generalized muscular weakness; fractures are frequent. SYN infantile osteomalacia, juvenile osteomalacia, rachitis.

5. **D.** *Ref:* TMD
   - Sudden infant death syndrome is sudden death of an infant younger than 1 year of age that remains unexplained after a thorough investigation, including a complete autopsy, examination of the death scene and review of the clinical history.

6. **C.** *Ref:* TMD
   - Vitamin D is necessary for the absorption of calcium and phosphorous from food in the small intestine. It is called the anti-rachitic vitamin because its deficiency interferes with calcium and phosphorous, which in turn causes rickets.

7. **D.** *Ref:* Harrison P–2375, HM P–249 & TMD
   - In children, prior to epiphyseal fusion, vitamin D deficiency results in growth retardation associated with an expansion of the growth plate known as Rickets.
   - Rickets occurs in growing children from 6 months to 2 years of age. The disease has the following lesions and clinical characterstics:
   - Skeletal changes: These are as under:
     1. Craniotabes is the earliest bony lesion occurring due to small round unossified areas in the membranous bones of the skull, disappearing within 12 months of birth. The skull looks square and box-like.
     2. Harrison's sulcus appears due to indrawing of soft ribs on inspirations.
     3. Rachitic rosary is a deformity of chest due to cartilaginous overgrowth at costochondral junction.
     4. Pigeon-chest deformity is the anterior protrusion of sternum due to action of respiratory muscles.
     5. Bow legs occur in ambulatory children due to weak bones of lower legs.
     6. Knock knees may occur due to enlarged ends of the femur, tibia and fibula.
     7. Lower epiphyses of radius may be enlarged.
     8. Lumbar lordosis is due to involvement of the spine and pelvis. – HM

- Rickets is a vitamin D deficiency in children that results in inadequate deposition of lime salts in developing cartilage and newly formed bone, causing abnormalities in the shape and structure of bones.

8. B. *Ref:* Harrison P–442, HM P–252, TMD

- Alcoholic patients with chronic thiamine deficiency may also have central nervous system (CNS) manifestations known as Wernicke's encephalopathy, consisting of horizontal nystagmus, ophthalmoplegia(due to weakness of one or more extraocular muscles), cerebellar ataxia, and mental impairment.
- Wernicke's encephalopathy occurs more often due to conditioned deficiencies such as in chronic alcoholism. It is characterised by degeneration of ganglia cells, focal demyelination and hemorrhage in the nuclei surrounding the region of ventricles and aqueduct. –HM
- Wernicke encephalopathy is associated with thiamine deficiency; usually associated with chronic alcoholism, gastric carcinoma, or hyperemesis gravidarum.

9. C. *Ref:* Harrison P–445 & TMD

- Actions of vitamin C include antioxidant activity, promotion of nonheme iron absorption, carnitine biosynthesis, the conversion of dopamine to norepinephrine, and the synthesis of many peptide hormones.
- Vitamin C is an ascorbic acid, a factor necessary for formation of collagen in connective tissues and essential in maintenance of integrity of intercellular cement in many tissues esp. capillary walls.

10. B. *Ref:* TMD

- Acrodermatitis enteropathica is a rare disease in children aged 3 weeks to 18 months that may be fatal if untreated. The genetically determined cause is mal-absorption of zinc.

11. D. *Ref:* Harrison P–469 & TMD

- Three key anthropometric measurements are important to evaluate the degree of obesity-weight, height, and waist circumference. The body mass index (BMI), calculated as weight (kg)/height (m)^2, or as weight (ibs)/ height (inches)^2 × 703, is used to classify weight status and risk of disease.
- An index for estimating obesity, obtained by dividing weight in kilograms by height in meters squared is called BMI. Age is important factor in interpreting these values because a high level in a young person is more likely to indicate obesity than an old man.

Thirteen

Preoperative Evaluation

QUESTIONS

1. Lumbar puncture is dangerous in:
   A. Subarachnoid haemorrhage
   B. Intracranial berry aneurysms
   C. Spinal cord tumours
   D. Intracranial tumours

ANSWERS AND EXPLANATIONS WITH REFERENCES

1. D. *Ref:* T.C.M.D

- Lumbar puncture is a puncture made by placing an aspiration needle into the subarachnoid space of the spinal cord, usually in the lumbar area at the level of the fourth intervertebral space. This procedure is done to inject an anesthetic solution, to measure the pressure of the cerebrospinal fluid (CSF), or to obtain a sample of CSF for determining its constituents (e.g., pathogens, blood, proteins, excess white blood cells). The information obtained is esp. helpful in diagnosing bacterial meningitis and central nervous system syphilis. SYN: spinal puncture.

Fourteen

Miscellaneous

QUESTIONS

1. Drug which is safe in pregnancy is:
A. Adenosine
B. Enalapril
C. Sodium nitroprusside
D. ACE receptor antagonist

2. Morphine for pain is not to be used in which of the following conditions:
A. Terminal cancer pain
B. Post operative pain
C. Biliary colic
D. Myocardial infarction

3. All of the following acts on cell membrane receptors except:
A. Factor X
B. Factor XI
C. Factor II
D. Factor VII

4. Reye's syndrome is caused by:
A. Mefenamic acid
B. Salycilates
C. Naproxen
D. Ibuprofen

5. Diagoxin levels are increased by addition of which of the following:
A. Phenytoin
B. Quinidine
C. Furesemide
D. Steroids

6. Most common tumor of infancy is:
A. Ameloblastoma
B. Hemangioma
C. Neuroblastoma
D. Retinoblastoma

7. Most of the neuroblastoma arises within:
   A. Abdomen
   B. Pelvis
   C. Adrenal gland
   D. Abdominal paravertebral autonomic ganglion

8. How much estrogen is present in oral contraceptive pill?
   A. More than 1 mgm
   B. Less than 50 micro gm
   C. Less than 50 nano gram
   D. More than 50 micro gm

ANSWERS AND EXPLANATIONS WITH REFERENCES

1. A. Ref: T.C.M.D.
- Adenosine is a nucleotide containing adenine and ribose.

2. C. Ref: T.C.M.D.
- Biliary colic is pain caused by the pressure or passing of gallstones.

3. B.

4. B. *Ref:* HM P–602 & T.C.M.D
- Reye's syndrome is defined as an acute postviral syndrome of encephalopathy and fatty change in the viscera. The syndrome may follow almost any known viral disease but is most common after influenza A or B and varicella. – HM
- Reye's syndrome is a syndrome first recognized in 1963, marked by acute encephalopathy and fatty infiltration of the liver and possibly of the pancreas, heart, kidney, spleen, and lymph nodes.

5. B. *Ref:* T.C.M.D.
- Quinidine sulfate is the sulfate of an alkaloid obtained

from cinchona bark a white crystalline substance with a bitter taste. It is used to regulate heart rhythm, esp. to prevent fibrillation.

6. **B.** *Ref:* COM P- 80 & TMD
   - Hemangioma is a tumor of dilated blood vessels. Hemangioma may be a congenital anomaly, in which proliferation of blood vessels leads to a mass that resembles a neoplasm. They arise in childhood and are found on the skin, in the scalp and within the connective tissue of mucous membra1ne. – COM
   - Hemangioma is a benign tumor of dilated blood vessels.

7. **A**. *Ref:* TMD
   - Neuroblastoma is a malignant hemorrhagic tumor composed principally of cells resembling neuroblasts that give rise to cell of the sympathetic system, esp. adrenal medulla.

8. **B.** *Ref:* Harrison P–2333 & TMD
   - Because of their ease of use and efficacy, oral contraceptive pill are the most widely used form of hormonal contraceptive pills.
   - The term contraceptive is any process, device, or, method that prevents conception. Estrogen is any naturals or artificial substance that induces estrus and the development of female sex characteristics.